Sexual H and the M

Guest Editor: John M Tomlinson

Series Editors: Margaret Rees and Tony Mander

The ROYAL
SOCIETY *of*
MEDICINE
PRESS *Limited*

BRITISH MEN~~OPAUSE SOCIETY~~
Meeting the Ch~~~~

© 2005 Royal Society of Medicine Press Ltd
Published by the Royal Society of Medicine Press Ltd
1 Wimpole Street, London W1G 0AE, UK
Tel: +44 (0) 20 7290 2921
Fax: +44 (0) 20 7290 2929
Email: publishing@rsm.ac.uk
Website: www.rsmpress.co.uk

The authors are responsible for the scientific content and for the views expressed, which are not necessarily those of the Royal Society of Medicine or of the Royal Society of Medicine Press Ltd or British Menopause Society Publications Ltd.

Although every effort has been made to ensure that, where provided, information concerning drug dosages or product usage has been presented accurately in this publication, the ultimate responsibility rests with the prescribing physician and neither the publisher nor the sponsor can be held responsible for errors or any consequences arising from the use of information contained herein.

British Library Cataloguing in Publication Data

A catalogue record for this book is available from the British Library
ISBN 1 85315 620 5

Distribution in Europe and Rest of World:
Marston Book Services Ltd
PO Box 269
Abingdon
Oxon OX14 4YN, UK
Tel: +44 (0) 1235 465500
Fax: +44 (0) 1235 465555
Email: direct.order@marston.co.uk

Distribution in the USA and Canada:
Royal Society of Medicine Press Ltd
c/o Jamco Distribution Inc.
1401 Lakeway Drive
Lewisville TX 75057, USA
Tel: +1 800 538 1287
Fax: +1 972 353 1303
Email: jamco@majors.com

Distribution in Australia and New Zealand:
Elsevier Australia
30–52 Smidmore Street
Marrickville NSW 2204
Australia
Tel: + 61 2 9517 8999
Fax: + 61 2 9517 2249
Email: service@elsevier.com.au

Designed and typeset by Phoenix Photosetting, Chatham, Kent

Printed and bound by Krips b.v., Meppel, The Netherlands

List of contents

About the editors

John Tomlinson was formerly senior partner in a four-partner undergraduate and postgraduate teaching practice in Alton, Hampshire, and was Honorary Senior Lecturer at the University of Southampton. He has run a men's health clinic at the Royal Hampshire County Hospital in Winchester, which he started in 1995 – as soon as it was possible to treat erectile dysfunction. He has also been interested in and taught on sexual and psychosexual problems for 25 years and edited the *ABC of Sexual Health*, the second edition of which has just been published.

Margaret Rees is a Medical Gynaecologist and Reader in Reproductive Medicine in the Nuffield Department of Obstetrics and Gynaecology, University of Oxford. She runs the menopause clinic in Oxford – one of the first founded in the UK. She is editor in chief of the *Journal of the British Menopause Society*, a trustee of the Sexual Dysfunction Association and an expert advisor to Women's Health Concern.

Tony Mander is a Consultant Gynaecologist, deputy editor of the *Journal of the British Menopause Society* and honorary clinical teacher in Obstetrics and Gynaecology at Manchester University. He is a member of the academic board, Royal Society of Medicine and an expert advisor to Women's Health Concern.

List of contributors

Walter Pierre Bouman
Consultant Psychiatrist-Sexologist for Older People, Mental Health Services for Older People, University Hospital, Nottingham, UK

Ailsa Gebbie
Consultant in Community Gynaecology, Lothian Primary Care NHS Trust, Family Planning and Well Woman Services, Edinburgh, UK

Clive Gingell
Consultant Urologist, Bristol, UK

Phillip Hodson
Psychotherapist, Fellow of the British Association for Counselling and Psychotherapy; in private practice, London, UK

Faryal Mahar
Specialist Registrar in Genitourinary Medicine, Department of Genitourinary Medicine, Radcliffe Infirmary, Oxford, UK

Margaret Ramage
Psychosexual Therapist, Wandsworth Primary Care Trust & Lambeth Primary Care Trust, London, UK

Jackie Sherrard
Consultant Physician, Department of Genitourinary Medicine, Radcliffe Infirmary, Oxford, UK

John M Tomlinson
Physician, Men's Health Clinic, Royal Hampshire County Hospital, Winchester; Clays Farm, East Worldham, Alton, UK

Gill Wakley
General Practitioner, Abergavenny, UK; Visiting Professor in Primary Care Development, Staffordshire University, UK

Rose Whiteley
Counsellor and Psychosexual Therapist in private practice, Bedforshire, UK

Kevan Wylie
Consultant in Sexual Medicine, Porterbrook Clinic, Royal Hallamshire Hospital, Sheffield, UK

Preface

Everyone hopes to enjoy good health for as long as possible. Sexual health is an integral component of wellbeing and many postmenopausal women have an increased sexual responsiveness as a result of a reduced fear of pregnancy, no longer having to use contraceptives, or the end of menstrual distress. On the other hand, older women may complain of dyspareunia, lack of or diminished sexual desire, difficulty becoming sexually aroused (either physically or psychologically), and difficulty achieving orgasm.

Understanding sexual problems involves many disciplines, including general practitioners, gynaecologists, genito-urinary physicians, geriatricians, clinical psychologists, and nurses both in primary and secondary care. During consultations female sexual problems may be mentioned briefly and apparently as an 'after thought' even though they are the main problem – being able to recognize these problems is an important part of the health professional's job. Because sexual health is very much a 'couple phenomenon', male problems must also be assessed. Treatment is not limited to pharmacotherapy but also includes various self-help methods.

During the peri-menopause women may falsely believe that they are infertile and an unplanned pregnancy is potentially disastrous – use of contraception is therefore essential. Traditionally, older people are not considered to be at risk of sexually transmitted infections, but several factors may predispose them to a higher infection rate and there may be a delay in symptom recognition. Women in the general population and health professionals must be made aware of this.

The aim of this book is to provide up-to-date information on female sexual dysfunction, male sexual problems, contraception in the peri-menopause and sexually transmitted diseases. Experts have written the chapters to provide an integrated and easy-to-read book for busy health professionals who deal with peri-menopausal and postmenopausal women. The further reading lists found at the end of each chapter are a selection of the most recent and relevant publications.

John M Tomlinson
Margaret Rees
Tony Mander

1 Keeping sex alive in later years

Walter Pierre Bouman

Introduction

Sexual intimacy and sexual activity is an important quality-of-life issue for everybody. The increase in life expectancy and the ever-growing population of older adults, particularly women, make discussion of sex and sexual health in this age group timely and topical.

Research shows predominantly negative attitudes to sexuality in older people, particularly among younger individuals. More recent work, however, suggests that some positive changes have occurred, and generally more positive attitudes towards ageing sexuality are being reported in the literature. This is likely to be a reflection of our societies' increasingly liberal attitude towards sexuality, together with the development of a consumer culture, with new opportunities and roles for older people.

Society's growing openness about sexual issues in the last decades, reflected in the publication of books as diverse as Alex Comfort's *The joy of sex*, Nancy Friday's *My secret garden* and *Forbidden flowers* and Jennifer and Laura Berman's *For women only*, have made many (older) women more comfortable with their own sexuality. Results of current multinational trials of sildenafil in women with sexual dysfunction are awaited eagerly and inevitably will raise the profile of female sexuality – in the same way as happened for men.

Myths regarding sexuality in older women

Many myths regarding sexuality exist in our society. A myth can be defined as an untrue idea or explanation that is often used to show disapproval.

Box 1.1 shows some myths described in both medical and fictional literature pertinent to sexuality in older women. Many more similar ones exist. It is important to note that we all hold myths regarding sexuality, which stem from transgenerational internalized social, political, religious, cultural and moral values. As health professionals, however, we have a duty to examine critically and evaluate our own sexual myths and ideally to dispel them.

Box 1.1

Sexual myths

- Sexual activity is only for those under thirty
- A woman's sex life ends with the menopause
- A sexually responsive woman can always be 'turned on' by her partner
- Nice decent women are not aroused by erotica

Facts about sexual activity in older women

To dispel the first myth, it is well established that women's sexual responsiveness increases with age, does not peak until their mid-thirties and continues throughout the lifecycle, with only slightly reduced interest and functioning in many women, except during or after illness and bereavement. It has consistently been shown that many post-menopausal women have an increased sexual responsiveness, which may be due to factors such as a reduced fear of pregnancy, no longer having to use contraceptives and the end of menstrual distress.

Early studies found that 47% of married women aged between 66 and 71 years are sexually active, and of those aged over 78 years, up to 29% are sexually active. The most current survey by the National Council on Aging and the American Association for Retired Persons showed that of 1000 men and women aged over 50 years, 60% were satisfied with their sex lives. Sixty-one percent reported that sex was as good or better than when they were young, and 70% had sex at least once a week. Of the participants in this survey who said their sex life was bland to non-existent, 34% mostly reported problems with illness, loss of a partner or drugs that robbed them of energy and enthusiasm for sexual activity. It is clear, however, that people who have been sexually active on a frequent basis throughout their life will show a lower rate of decline in activity with advancing years than those who have been less active.

Sexual physiology in older women

Explicit information about changes in sexual physiology with ageing can help eliminate false expectations. Many older adults are unaware of the normal age-related changes in sexual response that accompany ageing and are put off by changes in their own or their partner's sexual response.

For women, the menopause, which occurs on average at age 50 years, represents a clear marker of ageing. Menopausal symptoms may last for several years and may have an impact on women's sexuality in various ways.

Psychologically, the menopause may represent a point beyond which a woman feels she no longer can be, or should be, sexually attractive. Some women will experience a sense of loss about their childbearing years having come to an end. Even so, research suggests that the majority of women feel relief over the cessation of their periods and do not agree that they become less sexually attractive following the menopause.

Physically, irregular and sometimes heavy periods that finally stop altogether, hot flushes, severe night sweats and vaginal dryness can be highly disruptive to a sexual relationship. Painful uterine contractions at orgasm also seem to be more common after the menopause. The natural loss of collagen may result in the vagina becoming less elastic, particularly in those who are not sexually active.

Finally, stress incontinence is also associated with reduced oestrogen supplies and is yet another contribution to diminished sexual comfort for some older women.

Although this catalogue of decline may seem gloomy, it is important to realize that for most women this process is extremely gradual, allowing a woman to adjust to a less intense, but not necessarily less enjoyable, form of sexual activity.

Sexual problems in older women

In many respects, the sexual complaints of older women mirror those of their younger counterparts:

- lack of, or diminished, sexual desire
- difficulty becoming sexually aroused – either physically or psychologically
- difficulty achieving orgasm
- pain
- discomfort with sexual exchange, especially intercourse.

Dyspareunia is the most common sexual complaint of older women who seek gynaecological advice. Low-dose vaginal oestrogens, such as oestradiol and oestriol, are effective treatments.

In addition to these problems, women may mourn or regret changes in their body – its size, shape and firmness may differ significantly from the past. They also may complain about the changing body of their partner, the reduction in, or loss of, passion and attention given to emotional and sexual intimacy and changes in sexual urgency or intensity. Menopause, surgery and various losses – both psychological and physical – can exacerbate these complaints.

Sexuality in new and long-term relationships

It is not uncommon for couples of all ages to find themselves in a sexual and relationship stalemate. In many long-term relationships, predictability often replaces spontaneity, and sexual encounters may have become routine and perfunctory. Many couples feel some conflict between their needs for security and a stable relationship on the one hand and a desire for excitement and novelty on the other. Despite prevailing misconceptions, many older people indicate that they would enjoy greater sexual experimentation in their relationship. If people found sex to be a source of pleasure and gratification during early and middle adulthood, it probably will continue to be an important source of life satisfaction as they grow older.

However, the degree of congruence of sexual needs and expectations between a couple and their ability to communicate and compromise are critical components for marital and sexual adjustment and consequently overall satisfaction within the relationship.

Many older women may find themselves facing sexual activity with a new partner, which may be a very stressful prospect. Concerns about personal desirability, attractiveness and sex appeal, as well as the risks of acquiring sexually transmitted diseases, are often real and significant issues (Chapter 8). Advice on open communication and sexual education, particularly about practising safe sex, is paramount. It is perfectly acceptable for a woman to tell her partner how nervous she is: this may actually set a standard of open and positive communication that will not only make her feel safer but will also set the stage for enhanced sexual communication in general.

Nevertheless, it must be acknowledged that there remain many older women who grew up in a post-Victorian society and in traditional and religious households in which sexually proscriptive values and beliefs persist. For these women, sex is sanctioned primarily for procreation; sexual behaviours other than intercourse are considered unnatural, and masturbation is regarded as sinful. For such women, the opportunity to 'retire' from an active sexual life may be strongly anticipated and easily accepted.

How to help keep the sexuality of patients alive

Sexuality, in the old as well as the young, encompasses far more than a narrow focus on coital intercourse. There are many ways to keep sexuality alive. Even people who are completely satisfied with their sex life may want to use some creativity to enhance it. Box 1.2 gives a number of ways and techniques to enhance arousal and sexual pleasure – both for single women and women in a relationship. Some will appeal to many; others to a few.

Box 1.2

Ways and techniques to enhance arousal and sexual pleasure*

Good communication
- Keep the lines of communication in the relationship honest and open
- The best time to talk things through is probably not during sexual activity, as it is such an intimate and vulnerable setting
- A woman can provide positive feedback and encouragement when her partner is doing something that she finds pleasurable and stimulating
- Women who feel embarrassed about bringing up sexual issues with a partner may want to try introducing educational and erotic videos and books into their relationship

Prior to sexual activity
- Many women need to feel comfortable and safe before they can enjoy sex; the use of scents and lingerie can help
- Practising Kegel's exercises to strengthen pelvic floor muscles does not only help bladder control but can also lead to more intense orgasm and greater sexual pleasure
- Low-dose vaginal oestrogens can be used to improve dyspareunia

During sexual activity
- Using a gentle water-soluble lubricant may be enjoyable and add to sensitivity during sexual activity
- Baby oil and petroleum jelly, such as Vaseline, should be avoided, as they are not water soluble and tend to interfere with the vagina's natural protection against infection, as well as having the potential to break down the latex in condoms
- Sex aids, including vibrators, dildos and ticklers, as well as videos and sexy literature have the potential to improve the sex life
- Sexual activity is not just about intercourse. All couples, but especially older couples, can give each other sexual pleasure and orgasms through all sorts of activities that do not require erections or vaginal penetration – even when their range of motion has decreased. When the sexual activity is not orgasm focused, or intercourse focused, the act becomes much more a reflection of intimacy, connection, eroticism and arousal

---

*Based on recommendations made by Berman and Berman (2001) and Heiman and LoPiccolo (2001)

Institutional care for one or both partners may create additional barriers and problems that need to be overcome before conditions conducive to sexual intimacy can be met. Staff in care homes need education about the possible sexual needs of their residents, including ways of coping tactfully with the disinhibition that may accompany organic brain disease.

It is important that residential homes are sensitive to the fact that privacy and comfort are important. Bretschneider and McCoy reported that among healthy residents of retirement homes in California, 62% of men and 30% of women aged over 80 years had recently had sexual intercourse and that 82% and 64%, respectively, had had physical intimacy. Many care staff, however, often because of their own difficulty and embarrassment with the subject, assume that their elderly residents will be celibate. Discomfort with sexual issues may result in the use of ill-placed humour as a coping strategy, and staff therefore may treat the concept of relationships forming between or being maintained by elderly residents as both ridiculous and hilarious, adding to the pre-existing internalization of social disapproval and effectively incapacitating those in their care.

Conclusion

Giving patients 'permission' to learn about their own and their partner's sexuality and to experiment with new basic techniques is a powerful tool that clinicians must use. A satisfactory sex life contributes to good physical and mental health, as well as improving communication and the quality of the relationship.

Further reading

American Association for Retired Persons. *Healthy sexuality and vital aging*. Washington: American Association for Retired Persons, 1999.

Avis N. Women's perceptions of the menopause. *Eur Menopause J* 1996; 3: 80–4.

Berman J, Berman, L. *For women only. A revolutionary guide to reclaiming your sex life*. London: Virago Press, 2001.

Brecher E. *Love, sex and aging: a Consumer's Union survey*. Boston: Little Brown, 1984.

Bretchneider JG, McCoy NL. Sexual interest and behaviour in healthy 80–102 year olds. *Arch Sex Behav* 1988; 17: 109–29.

Dennerstein L, Dudley E, Burger H. Are changes in sexual functioning during midlife due to aging or menopause? *Fertil Steril* 2001; 76: 456–60.

Friday N. *My secret garden*. London: Quartes Books, 2001.

Friday N. *Forbidden flowers*. London: Arrow Books, 1994.

Heiman JR, LoPiccolo J. *Becoming orgasmic. A sexual and personal growth programme for women*. London: Judith Piatkus, 2001.

Leiblum SR. Taylor Seagraves R. Sex therapy with aging adults. In: Leiblum SR, Rosen RC, eds. *Principles and practice of sex therapy*. New York: Guilford Press, 2000.

May K, Riley A. Sexual function after 60. *J Br Menopause Soc* 2002; **8**: 112–14.

Milsom I. Symptoms, diagnosis and treatment of vaginal atrophy. *J Br Menopause Soc* 2002; **8**: 115–6.

Morley JE, Kaiser FE. Female sexuality. *Med Clin North Am* 2003; **87**: 1077–90.

Murgatroyd M. Sexual needs of elderly people in residential care. *Br J Sex Med* 1998; **21**: 4.

Öberg P, Tornstam L. Attitudes toward embodied old age among Swedes. *Int J Aging Hum Dev* 2003; **56**: 133–53.

Oppenheimer C. Sexuality in old age. In: Jacoby R, Oppenheimer C, eds. *Psychiatry in the elderly*. Oxford: Oxford University Press, 2002.

Suckling J, Lethaby A, Kennedy R. Local oestrogen for vaginal atrophy in postmenopausal women. *Cochrane Database Syst Rev* 2003; **(4)**: CD001500.

Verwoerdt A, Pfeiffer E, Wang HS. Sexual behavior in senescence: changes in sexual activity and interest of aging men and women. *J Geriatr Psychiatry* 1969; **2**: 163–80.

2 Female sexual dysfunction and menopause

Margaret Ramage

Introduction
Models of the female sexual response
Causes of female sexual dysfunction
Female sexual dysfunction
Conclusion

Introduction

The menopause is a time when previously unacknowledged sexual difficulties become harder to deny, when physical changes give rise to sexual problems and when the end of fertility brings the whole matter of women's sexuality into high relief. Some women see this period as an opportunity to give up an activity that may never have been particularly enjoyable or satisfying, while others feel that, with children away from home and no risk of pregnancy, a new sexual relationship can develop. There seems to be some pressure from the media for women to remain sexually active and attractive, when in truth desire and enjoyment may have gone.

Whatever the issue for any individual, frequently there is some difficulty in communicating the problem to a professional. Without sensitive yet direct questioning, sexual problems and concerns may not be revealed, and help may be needed to find words to express what can feel impossible to say. Because of shame and a lack of appropriate language in which to describe sexual matters, a woman may complain of vague symptoms that are confusingly described and bewildering to the clinician.

Sexual problems may be the first indicator of underlying illness, a sign of a deteriorating marital relationship, a symptom caused by oestrogen deficiency or a manifestation of the woman's attempts to address aging and all that it brings. It is up to the clinician to understand and uncover what may be going on for the woman – and that is a complicated task. Currently, there is some pressure (often from the partner rather than from the woman herself) for a quick treatment that will answer all problems. This compounds the challenge facing the clinician, as there are a number of mechanical and pharmacological aids to choose from, but these have given rise to concerns about the risk of overmedicalization of sexuality or, conversely, failure to identify underlying illness.

Models of the female sexual response

Masters and Johnson elaborated the first model of female sexual response on the basis of a study of 694 volunteers aged over 11 years of both sexes. They proposed a four-phase linear, sequential and incremental model of the human response cycle (see Figure 2.1). This was the EPOR model:

- excitation (E) stimuli from somatogenic or psychogenic sources raise sexual tensions
- plateau (P) sexual tensions intensified
- orgasmic (O) involuntary pleasurable climax
- resolution (R) dissipation of sexual tensions.

Helen Kaplan, a sex therapist from New York, proposed that a desire phase (D) should exist before the E phase – the DEOR model (Figure 2.1). Levin

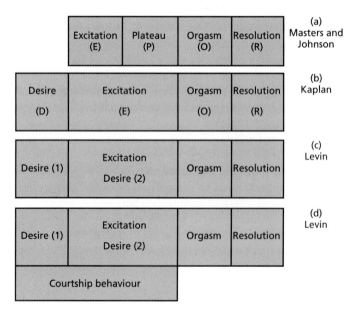

Figure 2.1 The development of the four-phase human sexual response model from: (a) the original EPOR model of Masters and Johnson (1966) through (b) the DEOR model of Kaplan (1979), with the added desire phase and the dropped plateau (P-phase) replaced by the extended excitation or E-phase, to (c) the newer female model of a split desire phase into the original desire phase 1 (D1, spontaneous, endogenous) and the new desire phase 2 (D2, activated by excitation). Adapted from Levin (2000) and Levin (2001)

then questioned the location of the desire phase in the sequential DEOR model and proposed two types: D1 (spontaneous) and D2 (activated by excitation). Courtship behaviour that begins the initiation of sexual activity is also difficult to position in regard to the DEOR model.

Concerns are that these models overemphasize the physiological aspects of sexuality at the expense of the emotional aspects. There is also an assumption that male and female sexualities are parallel and similar. Basson thus developed an alternative model, in which the power behind the cycle is the couple's emotional intimacy, and this power or 'motor' may be enhanced or diminished by the experience itself, see Figure 2.2.

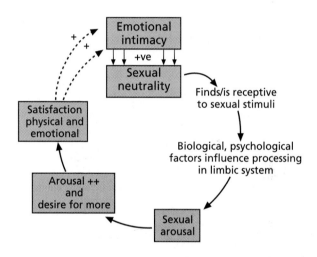

Figure 2.2 Female sexual response. Adapted from Basson (2002)

Causes of female sexual dysfunction

The Working Group for a New View of Women's Sexual Problems compiled a comprehensive overview of causes of female sexual dysfunction (FSD), which is summarized in Box 2.1. Any life changing events, such as losses, abuses and lifestyle changes, may give rise to sexual difficulties at any age – not only during the menopausal years.

Box 2.1

Working Group for a New View of Women's Sexual Problems: overview of causes of female sexual dysfunction

Sexual problems due to sociocultural, political or economic factors

Such problems include:
- Ignorance and anxiety due to inadequate sex education, poor access to health services and lack of language
- Sexual avoidance or distress due to perceived inability to meet cultural norms and shame about body, sexual attractiveness or sexual identity
- Inhibitions due to conflict between the sexual norms of subculture and those of the dominant culture
- Lack of interest, fatigue or lack of time due to family and work obligations

Sexual problems relating to partner and relationship

Such problems include:
- Inhibition, avoidance or distress arising from betrayal, dislike or fear of partner, partner's abuse, power imbalance or poor communication
- Discrepancies in desire for sexual activity or preferences
- Difficulty in communicating preferences or initiating, pacing or shaping activities
- Loss of sexual interest as a result of conflicts or traumatic experiences, such as infertility or the death of a child
- Inhibitions in arousal or spontaneity due to partner's health or sexual problems

Sexual problems due to psychological factors

Such problems include:
- Sexual aversion, mistrust or inhibition of sexual pleasure due to past abuse, problems with attachment, depression or anxiety
- Sexual inhibition due to fear of sexual acts or their consequences – for example, pain during intercourse, pregnancy, a sexually transmitted disease, loss of partner or loss of reputation

Sexual problems due to medical factors, such as pain or lack of physical response, despite a good relationship, adequate knowledge and positive attitudes

Such problems arise from:
- Medical conditions that affect neurological, neurovascular, circulatory, endocrine or other systems of the body
- Pregnancy, sexually transmitted diseases or other sex-related conditions
- Side effects of drugs, medications or medical treatments
- Iatrogenic conditions

Female sexual dysfunction

The classification of female sexual dysfunction is problematic, and the attempts of the *International classification of disease (tenth revision)* (ICD 10) (WHO, 1999) and the *Diagnostic and statistical manual of mental disorders – fourth revision* (DSM 1V) (American Psychiatric Association 1994) received criticism from the Working Group for a New View of Women's Sexual Problems. The two main complaints are that both classifications follow the human sexual response cycle proposed by Masters and Johnson and later elaborated by Kaplan.

In 2000, the International Consensus Development Conference on Female Sexual Dysfunction provided a classification system suitable for clinical diagnosis and research purposes, which addressed these problems (see Table 2.1). The consensus definitions provide a common language with which women and clinicians can communicate with each other and a basis for further research in to prevalence, aetiology and therapy. One of the major changes in the classification schema was to add 'personal distress' as a criterion of the diagnosis.

Menopausal and ageing women have numerous emotional challenges to deal with and the impact of these on both the emotional climate and the relationship is almost inevitable, so it is not surprising that the incidence of all sexual problems increases in this age group (Castelo-Branco *et al* 2003). The categories of women's sexual problems as they commonly present are outlined below, but the clinician may need to bear in mind that the presenting problem is very often not the real one.

Problems with desire and arousal

Recent studies have identified that desire and arousal are inextricably intertwined much of the time, and physiological changes of arousal, such as vaginal lubrication and pelvic engorgement, often are unnoticed by the woman. This confirms what many women know – that they do not feel the need to initiate sexual activity but can enjoy it when it happens. As oestrogen levels drop and vaginal dryness and discomfort become more prevalent, desire and arousal response are likely to be affected. The lack of any feeling of desire is more common in menopausal women, but it does not signal the end of sexual pleasure. When a woman or her partner perceives a change in her level of sexual desire or arousal as a problem, it may require attention. For some women it is 'just how it is' and they are quite philosophical about it, but the partner may be pressurizing her to change. Discrepancy in desire levels between partners can lead to much anguish, with the woman often labelled as 'the problem', whether her desire is the higher or the lower!

Table 2.1

Consensus classification system. Adapted from Basson (2000)

Classification	Definition
I Sexual desire disorders	
A Hypoactive sexual desire disorder (HSDD)	The persistent or recurrent deficiency (or absence) of sexual fantasies/thoughts and/or desire for or receptivity to sexual activity, which causes personal distress
B Sexual aversion disorder (SAD)	The persistent or recurrent phobic aversion and avoidance of sexual contact with a sexual partner, which causes personal distress
II Sexual arousal disorders	The persistent or recurrent inability to attain or maintain sufficient sexual excitement, causing personal distress, which may be expressed as a lack of subjective excitement, or genital (lubrication/swelling) or other somatic responses
III Orgasmic disorder	The persistent or recurrent difficulty, delay in or absence of attaining orgasm after sufficient sexual stimulation and arousal, which causes personal distress
IV Sexual pain disorders	
A Dyspareunia	The recurrent or persistent genital pain associated with sexual intercourse
B Vaginismus	The recurrent or persistent involuntary spasm of the musculature of the outer third of the vagina, which interferes with vaginal penetration and causes personal distress
C Noncoital sexual pain disorders	Recurrent or persistent genital pain induced by noncoital sexual stimulation

Each of the categories above is subtyped on the basis of the medical history, physical examination and laboratory tests as: (A) lifelong versus acquired; (B) generalized versus situational or (C) aetiology (organic, psychogenic, mixed or unknown)

Problems with orgasm

Some women develop orgasmic ability over time and with experimentation; others – about 10% – do not experience orgasm at all. A woman may be anorgasmic, or pre-orgasmic, in which case she would believe she has never experienced an orgasm or climax, or she may have ceased being orgasmic for a number of reasons – medical illness among them. Male partners often are more troubled by a lack of orgasm than the woman herself, drawing parallels between male and female sexualities. A man may see it as a failure or lack of prowess on his behalf, while the woman is satisfied with sex as it is. Reduction in the intensity of orgasm is common during and after the menopause.

Aversion, phobia, and 'sexual anorexia'

These three presentations of sexual avoidance may occur at any time in life but are more common in younger women. Strong feelings of revulsion at the prospect of sexual activity are typical of sexual aversion and may result from early childhood events or later problems, frequently with the theme of disgust, humiliation and shame. Sexual phobia, or fear of sexual contact, is a common response to earlier trauma, abuse or violation. The sexual anorexic may feel willing and want to be sexual but cannot allow herself to proceed when in the sexual encounter. She may have low self-esteem, and issues of upbringing are likely antecedents. In all three presentations, the woman may be puzzled at her reactions and go to great lengths to avoid being in sexual situations. Some are able to overcome their reluctance from time to time – usually with the help of alcohol and other drugs. All may have familial and relationship disturbances underlying the sexual symptom and are likely to require psychotherapeutic help.

Painful sex

Pain that occurs in the absence of any infection or inflammation may indicate insufficient vaginal lubrication or incomplete arousal, so that the inner part of the vagina does not expand to make space for penetration. Lubricants and topical hormone treatments are available for this, if indicated. Alternatively, vulvodynia, which causes exquisite pain to the touch, could be present, and this would require gynaecological assessment and possibly medication. In some circumstances, psychotherapeutic help is indicated.

Vaginismus

This is painful involuntary spasm of the pubococcygeus muscle that renders penetration either very painful or impossible. It is usually caused by fear of the pain of penetration and responds well to a combined physical and psychological intervention – similar to that described by Bergson and Lord (2003), including the use of vaginal trainers, which are graded plastic rods inserted in to the vagina by the woman for gradual dilation at her own pace and ability. When vaginismus occurs in later life, the dynamics of the relationship and the woman's psychological state are likely to need very thorough assessment. A deteriorating marital relationship may be manifested by this condition.

Conclusion

When a woman complains of a sexual difficulty, it is usually in the hope that something can be done, and she may expect to be referred for couple or sexual therapy, for further investigations or to other specialist consultation. It is useful for clinicians to have some knowledge of local services and specialists.

Further reading

American Psychiatric Association. *Diagnostic and statistical manual of mental disorders – fourth edition* (DSM-IV). Washington: American Psychiatric Press, 1994.

d'Ardenne P, Morod D. *The counselling of couples in healthcare settings: a handbook for clinicians*. London: Whurr, 2003.

Basson R. Rethinking low sexual desire in women. *Br J Obstet Gynaecol* 2002; **109**: 357–63.

Basson R. Women's sexual dysfunctions: revised and expanded. *Sex Relat Therap* 2004; **19 (Suppl 1)**: 34, S31.

Basson R, Leiblum S, Brotto L, *et al.* Definitions of women's sexual dysfunction reconsidered: advocating expansion and revision. *J Psychosom Obstet Gynaecol* 2003; **24**: 221–9.

Basson R, Berman J, Burnett A, *et al.* Report of the international consensus development conference on female sexual dysfunction: definitions and classifications. *J Urol* 2000; **163**: 888–93.

Bergson S, Lord M-J. The integration of pelvi-perineal re-education and cognitive-behavioural therapy in the multidisciplinary treatment of pelvic pain disorders. *Sex Relat Therap* 2003; **18**: 135–41.

Castelo-Branco C, Blumel JE, Araya H, *et al.* Prevalence of sexual dysfunction in a cohort of middle-aged women: influences of menopause and hormone replacement therapy. *J Obstet Gynaecol* 2003; **23**: 426–30.

Hawton K. *Sex therapy: a practical guide*. Oxford: Oxford University Press, 1985.

Kaplan HS. *Disorders of sexual desire*. New York: Brunner/Mazel, 1979.

Kashak E, Tiefer L, eds. *A new view of women's sexual problems*. Binghampton: Haworth Press, 2001: 5–7.

Levin RJ. Sexual desire and the deconstruction and reconstruction of the human female sexual response model of Masters & Johnson. In: Everaerd W, Laan E, Both S, eds. *Sexual appetite, desire and motivation: energetics of the sexual system*. Amsterdam: Royal Netherlands Academy of Arts and Sciences, 2001.

Levin RJ. Normal sexual function. In: Gelder MG, Lopez-Ibor JJ, Andreasen N, eds. *New Oxford textbook of psychiatry. Volume 1*. Oxford: Oxford University Press, 2000: 875–82.

Masters WH, Johnson V. *Human sexual response*. Boston: Little Brown, 1966.

Moynihan R. The making of a disease: female sexual dysfunction. *BMJ* 2003; **326**: 45–7.

Ramage M. Female sexual dysfunction. *Psychiatry* 2004; **3**: 16–22.

World Health Organization. *International statistical classification of diseases and related health problems (tenth revision)*. Geneva: World Health Organization, 1999.

3 Recognizing female sexual problems

Gill Wakley

Introducing the subject of sex
The consultation
The examination
Investigations
Presentation of sexual problems
Illness or treatment affecting sexuality
Types of problems presented
Conclusion

Introducing the subject of sex

The prevalence of sexual problems in the general population has been investigated by several community studies. A study in several general practices in the UK found rates of 44% for men and 36% for women. Sexual problems increase in men as they grow older, but there seems little evidence that this generally occurs in women. Social and physiological factors seem to have more influence on women's sexual functioning. Health professionals in primary care need to become more aware of the overlap between sexual dysfunction and the mental or physical ill health that affects large numbers of their patients, and careful proactive enquiry may prevent avoidable errors.

If you miss sexual dysfunction, you will give the wrong advice or treatment – such as referring a patient to a psychiatrist about depression and anxiety when the problem is dyspareunia. Unnecessary treatment can be avoided – for example, by understanding exactly what a patient means when she complains of 'cystitis' when in fact the problem is atrophic vulvo-vaginitis.

The importance of preventing sexually transmitted infections means that a change of sexual partners at the mean age for divorce (around 40 years of age) should remind health professionals to ask about sexual behaviour – see Chapter 8.

Be aware that patients may not take important treatments, such as antidepressants, because they affect their sex life.

The consultation

Sexual activity is usually a private concern often alluded to by innuendo and non-verbal signals. Talking about sex may be accompanied by reticence and embarrassment on the part of the health professional or the patient. Elicit the patient's problem by using your consultation skills (Box 3.1). If you ask a lot of questions you obtain many answers – but you may not hear what the problem is, because you have not allowed the patient to tell you. Patients often have within themselves the information that can help them resolve their sexual problems in a way that will suit them best. The health professional does not need to be an expert at sexual problems – just an expert at helping patients to find the solution.

Box 3.1

Consultation skills

- Illustrate or interpret how the patient may relate to others by seeing how the patient makes you feel
- Notice and interpret non-verbal communication
- Accept not being able to give an 'expert' answer
- Recognize your own biases and prejudices
- Have some knowledge of sexual functioning and emotional development
- Use the physical examination as an exploration of both the emotional and physical factors
- Give advice or reassurance only when you are sure you understand what the problem is for the patient
- Recognize when to refer elsewhere or suggest other avenues of help
- Limit offers of help when the patient is not making progress

---

The examination

Health professionals are very privileged to be able to look at the bodies of their patients. Listen and observe during the physical examination; it is not just to find or exclude physical abnormalities. Offering to examine a patient can be very helpful (see Table 3.1). Notice if you are avoiding doing a physical examination and consider who (the patient or you) is afraid of what? Offer a chaperone and respect the patient's wishes. Explain exactly what you are doing during the examination and why it is being undertaken. The patient should be quite clear about its normality or otherwise as you proceed and should understand why you are doing each part. Patients can misunderstand physical examination unless you communicate the reasons and the findings in the context of the problem. Reassure the patient that the examination will stop if they find it painful or distressing or if they ask you to stop.

Table 3.1

Female examination

Part of examination	Checkpoints
General inspection	• Check for mental distress or abnormality • Notice development of secondary sexual characteristics • Exclude hirsutism or other signs of virilization • Differentiate breathlessness due to respiratory disease when undressing or talking (which may limit the ability to be active during sexual activity) from acute anxiety
Cardio-vascular	• Check blood pressure, peripheral pulses and other signs of atherosclerosis or raised lipid levels (although these may be of uncertain aetiology in arousal disorders in women)
Musculoskeletal	• Osteoarthritis of the hips and back pain are common difficulties in older women and may be a severe physical barrier to intercourse
Nervous system	• Notice loss of sensation or reflexes in the perineal area; this is rare but may occur in patients with multiple sclerosis or spinal nerve damage
Abdominal	• Look for evidence of abdominal surgery and ask the patient about any scars, as the emotions expressed about them may be relevant and extensive pelvic surgery may damage pelvic nerves • Remember that irritable bowel syndrome, with pain from pressure on the distended or tender gut, is a common cause of dyspareunia
Genital	• Note and discuss with the patient the appearance of the genitals and look for lichen sclerosis • Assess for urinary stress incontinence if indicated by the history • A bimanual digital examination can confirm or exclude pain (such as bladder or ovarian pain produced by coital thrusting) and detect vaginismus. Pain-free digital examination when the complaint is dyspareunia is particularly helpful • Assess for adequate oestrogenization • Take swabs if there is discharge or irritation • Assess for gynaecological abnormalities such as fibroids or ovarian cysts

Investigations

Be guided by the history and examination. You would not want to check levels of follicle-stimulating hormone (FSH) to confirm the menopause if a woman aged 55 years has had no periods for four years. Sometimes, however, you need to do blood tests so that the woman can move away from the idea that she simply has a hormonal or physical problem that can be cured by medication, towards a more holistic view of the problem.

Presentation of sexual problems

Sexual problems may be:

- discovered as part of an ongoing illness, as a side-effect of treatment or as the result of disability
- presented openly
- presented after the patient has tried you out with a related (or even unrelated) complaint
- hidden by a psychosomatic complaint.

Illness or treatment affecting sexuality

Loss of interest in sexual activity while a person is ill is common. Be cautious in laying the blame in this direction – it may be a false clue or a source of false assumptions. For some couples, sexual activity is an important and essential reaffirmation of their love for each other, even when terminally ill.

Types of problems presented

The International Consensus Development Conference on Female Sexual Dysfunction produced a classification system (see Chapter 2) that often divides problems into:

- decreased or absent sexual desire (loss of libido)
- arousal disorders
- lack or loss of orgasm
- painful intercourse
- others, such as gender confusion and paraphilias (abnormal sexual activity that is socially prohibited).

In the real world, these categories often overlap, and one may cause the other. For example, painful intercourse is likely to lead to avoidance of sexual activity and anticipation of pain leads to lack of arousal, loss of orgasm and an increased chance of pain occurring.

Loss of desire

Loss of desire is the most common complaint in women but is a spectrum of disorders. The complaint may have always been present and may not really be a loss but a lack of desire for sexual activity. It may represent inhibition – a repression of sexual thoughts due to feelings of being too young (whatever the chronological age) or too pure (sex is dirty or unsuitable in some way) or sex being forbidden (by upbringing or religious taboo). It may represent a lack of compatibility between the expectations of the couple, either real or due to beliefs in myths.

Life events have a powerful effect on sexual functioning, and sexual problems are more likely at critical times. Looking at the circumstances of the difficulty for that couple or individual helps them to make sense of the situation and what they might do to modify or remedy the underlying causes. Sometimes the cause may be loss of attraction for, or even dislike of, the partner. Relationship therapy may be an option for motivated couples, but sometimes the patient just needs to come to terms with the realization that the partnership has to end. More often, a combination of several small adjustments in attitudes, thought patterns, assumptions or behaviour can be made by an individual or a couple to help the complainant move towards a resolution or acceptance of the problem.

Lack or loss of arousal

Lack of knowledge about the physiological changes that occur during arousal is still surprisingly common, perhaps because these changes are much less obvious in women. Such changes occur less well with diminution of the level of hormones with declining ovarian function. The plumping up of the tissues of the vulval fold and around the vagina, the pulling up of the uterus and ovaries and the variations in amount and timing of lubrication often require explicit explanation and discussion. Recommendation of a book can be helpful. The inhibition or enhancement of these changes by emotional states may be affected by many of the same factors mentioned above for desire.

Lack or loss of orgasm

Lack of orgasm is more common in women than in men. It may occur in those who have difficulty in showing their emotions, perhaps due to fear of a loss of control, or in those who are overcontrolling for some psychological gain. Other causes that can often be forgotten are antidepressant or antipsychotic drug treatment or neurological damage.

Orgasmic dysfunction in women often is linked to myths about the responsibility of the male partner to be able to produce orgasm 'for the woman'. Fears or inhibitions about masturbation may have prevented a woman from discovering how to produce an orgasm, or she may have been unable to transfer this experience to heterosexual activity.

Painful intercourse

Keep in mind that pain may not just arise from the genital area. Pain from any cause, such as osteoarthritis of the hip, may be inhibitory, especially if increased by sexual activity. Taking pain relief beforehand, or altering positions, in those with chronic painful conditions may make a considerable difference.

Vaginal fantasies

Some women fear that intercourse will cause pain, damage or bleeding. Men also have fantasies about the vagina. These may prevent erection, cause loss of erection when approaching the vagina or prevent ejaculation. Never jump to conclusions about other people's fantasies on the basis of what you have heard from others or what you might have within yourself. Expert guesses prevent patients explaining or exploring their own fantasies.

Sexual dysfunction following childbirth

Often patients date their sexual dysfunction to the birth of a baby. Remember that other changes may have been taking place at the same time – moving house, separation or loss of parents, loss of job or status, etc. Problems may have existed before but had been tolerated because of the desire for a baby or an expectation that all would be solved by the birth.

Male problems

Women may avoid intercourse because of concerns about erectile dysfunction or may not be able to cope with thinking they are unattractive or rejected. Couples may not be able to discuss or contemplate alternatives to penetrative sexual activity. Premature or retarded ejaculation may lead to a feeling of dissatisfaction by the woman. Retrograde ejaculation may be misunderstood as a failure or rejection (See Chapter 9).

Sexual violence

The realization that a woman has experienced sexual violence may emerge at any time but particularly at times of emotional crisis or when they have a genital examination. It may underlie sexual problems or relationship difficulties. Health practitioners have to deal with this difficult subject at the time it is revealed or risk the woman assuming that it is too terrible to hear.

Conclusion

A skilled doctor or nurse can manage most sexual problems in primary care. Consider referral if the patient or couple want this, wish to discuss the sexual dysfunction with someone not known to them, or have a problem that is beyond your competence that requires specialized or lengthy treatment for which facilities are not available in primary care.

Further reading

Balint M. *The doctor, his patient and the illness.* London: Pitman, 1964.

Barrett G, Pendry E, Peacock J, *et al.* Women's sexual health after childbirth. *Br J Obstet Gynaecol* 2000; **107**: 186–95.

Basson R, Berman J, Burnett A, *et al.* Report of the international consensus development conference on female sexual dysfunction: definitions and classifications. *J Urol* 2000; **163**: 888–93.

Cooper E, Guillebaud J. *Sexuality and disability – a guide for everyday practice.* Oxford: Radcliffe Medical Press, 1999.

Dunn KM, Jordan K, Croft PR, Assendelft WJJ. Systematic review of prevalence studies of common sexual problems. *J Sex Marit Therap* 2002; **28**: 399–422.

Dunn KM, Croft PR, Hackett GI. Sexual problems: a study of prevalence and need for health care in the general population. *Fam Pract* 1998; **15**: 519–24.

Guyatt GH, Haynes RB, Jaeschke RZ, *et al.* Users' guides to the medical literature: XXV. Evidence-based medicine: principles for applying the users' guides to patient care. Evidence-Based Medicine Working Group. *JAMA* 2000; **284**: 1290–6.

Haidet P, Paterniti DA. 'Building' a history rather than 'taking' one: a perspective on information sharing during the medical interview. *Arch Intern Med* 2003; **163**: 1134–40.

Laumann E, Park A, Rosen R. Sexual dysfunction in the United States, prevalence and predictors. *JAMA* 1999; **281**: 537–44.

Nazareth I, Boynton P, King M. Problems with sexual function in people attending London general practitioners: cross sectional study. *BMJ* 2003: **327**: 423–30.

Neighbour R. *The inner consultation.* Newbury: Petroc Press, 1999.

Ryan L, Hawton K. Female dyspareunia. *BMJ* 2004; **328**: 1357.

Skrine R. *Blocks & freedoms in sexual life.* Oxford: Radcliffe Medical Press, 1997.

Stewart E, Spencer P. *The V book.* London: Judy Piatkus Publishers, 2002.

Tomlinson JM, ed. *ABC of sexual health.* Oxford: Blackwell/BMJ Books, 2005.

Thompson D. 'Disabled people aren't interested in sex …' *J Fam Plann Reprod Health Care* 2003; **29**: 125–6.

Wakley G, Chambers R. *Sexual health matters in primary care.* Oxford: Radcliffe Medical Press, 2002.

Wakley G, Cunnion M, Chambers R. *Sexual health advice.* Oxford: Radcliffe Medical Press, 2003.

4 Taking a sexual history

John M Tomlinson

Introduction
Making the patient comfortable
Finding out the problem
Content of the history
Agreeing a management plan
Conclusion

Introduction

Taking a sexual history frequently bothers doctors and nurses because its introduction into the medical teaching curriculum is relatively recent and consultation time in primary and secondary care is limited. Doctors and nurses may be embarrassed about asking intimate questions or feel the patient may be embarrassed. The whole idea may make them so uncomfortable that they deal with it by:

- ignoring it completely
- brushing aside a patient's attempts to talk about a sexual problem
- medicalizing the answers to make themselves uninvolved and to feel safe – often to the patient's confusion.

Making the patient comfortable

As has been said in other chapters, the ability to take a good sexual history at the appropriate moment is essential, and to get the most important information, the patient should be made as comfortable and relaxed as possible. Various interview techniques can be used to help patients relax more quickly; most are used by many doctors intuitively. They include the manner of greeting a patient, seeing that the patient is seated comfortably and ensuring privacy and freedom from interruption (especially in a hospital clinic). A seat placed at the side of the desk provides a greater opportunity to observe the patient's body language, as well as being a more friendly arrangement.

- Greet the patient warmly – by name if possible and, if she is an older woman, by her title: Mrs, Miss, Dr, etc (many younger women, however, prefer to be greeted with first name or first and surname alone). Men find it easier to shake hands on first meeting, most women do not. Do whatever feels comfortable
- Look for body language, such as physical signs of nervousness and embarrassment – a flushed neck, nervous hand movements, whether the patient is relaxed and comfortably seated or is sat on the edge of the chair and whether the handbag, briefcase or shopping bag is put aside or defensively kept on the lap.
- Do not ask a patient questions, especially personal ones, when she is lying on a couch and you are standing beside her. She will feel very vulnerable and at a great disadvantage to have you looming over her.

Finding out the problem

When you start to ask a patient personal questions, it would be tactful to say you hope she does not mind being asked for some personal details. If the doctor or nurse is male, he will take a history from a male patient differently than from a woman patient, and the use of colloquialisms may be sex specific. When discussing a woman's periods, for example, common parlance can be used woman to woman, but its use sits very uneasily coming from a man (especially as he may get the terms wrong). Keep language simple and try not to use medical terms as the patient may not be sure what you mean. Judge how to talk to the patient by her age, class, culture and religion – for it is possible to be unintentionally offensive.

- Do not be judgemental of older women and men, particularly of their sexual habits.
- Remember that an older woman can be quite unnecessarily ashamed of having to ask for advice – so be unfazed and be gentle.
- Patients often have difficulty starting a conversation and are vague and circumlocutory. Pick up clues and clarify them. 'Sore down below' can mean anything – a discharge, warts, dyspareunia, a prolapse or a variety of other problems. Try and find out precisely what the patient is talking about before you examine her.
- Ask open questions such as 'How can I help you?' or 'How much of a bother is this?' rather than 'Are you having trouble with your periods?', which elicits a yes or no. 'Tell me what problems you are having' allows a woman to tell the story in her own words.
- If the patient asks you a question, a useful stratagem is often to reply with another question in the appropriate circumstances. For example, if the

patient asks, 'Do those blood pressure tablets you prescribed have any side-effects?', the doctor could answer medically and list a few of the most common side-effects, but a more effective way is to say, 'What sort of side-effects are you thinking about?' The patient will then respond 'Well, I seem to . . .', and out come the worries.

- Be careful not to jump in and come to the wrong conclusions. If a patient says, 'I'm having trouble sleeping at nights', it may or may not be due to her partner's (or her own) nocturia, but the patient's partner may well have erectile dysfunction and she is lying awake worrying about what is happening to their relationship. Giving her a sleeping pill would be inappropriate.

- Do not forget the value of silence. Most of us find it difficult to allow silences to fall, and we tend to jump in and fill the gap. During that silence, however, the patient is formulating her thoughts, and her mind will be busy. If you wait long enough, she will tell you. If you cut in, you will distract her and lose what may be very helpful information.

While you are taking a history, be aware of what Desmond Morris calls postural echo. This is a fascinating feature that will tell you when the patient is fully at ease. If she is, she will sit in an exact mirror image of you – whether with ankles crossed or arms folded, leaning an elbow on the side of the desk, mirroring your position in your chair, mirroring the position of your hands, whether touching the face or with fingers interlinked. It's a valuable clue, and can be used to make someone feel easier, especially if you adopt her position in reverse.

Repetition of the last word or phrase the patient has said, especially an emotive one, is a technique to get her to expand on what she is trying to say. It is used very commonly in everyday conversation without realizing it, but when used deliberately, it can be a very powerful tool to get history that would not normally be elicited. For example:

'Doctor, I think I need a check up.'
'Yes, of course. It's quite a time since the last one. Let me start with your blood pressure…'

Compare this with:

'Doctor, I think I need a check up.'
'Check up?'
'Yes, I keep getting these heavy periods.'
'Periods?'
'Yes, well, could I possibly have cancer?'
'Cancer?'
'I feel terrible. I'm tired, I'm flooding all the time and my mother had cancer of the womb.'

When to stop

It is also valuable to know when to stop asking questions. If you notice the patient becoming more uncomfortable, fidgeting, flushing and making awkward movements, stop, because she is probably finding your queries intrusive. Change the subject and allow her to reintroduce the topic if she becomes more relaxed. A bolder patient will often ask you why you are asking her these questions and you must have a good explanation. We must be very careful not to ask questions just to satisfy our own personal curiosity.

Content of the history

Although a joint interview with both partners is ideal for many sexual problems, the majority of patients prefer to see the doctor or nurse on their own in the first instance, especially if a discharge or possible sexually transmitted infection is involved.

Social history

If the problem turns out to be one where some discussion of the patient's relationship with her partner is required, ask her if she would like to bring him in (or her – don't automatically assume a partnership is heterosexual). Taking a social history before asking about the medical side gives the patient time to talk about home and children as well as her job and helps to put her medical problems into perspective.

Medical history

Ask about:

- the severity of the symptoms and their duration
- her relationship, its duration and the sex of her partner, with details of any possible cultural or religious differences
- the type of intercourse – vaginal, oral or anal (11.3% of women aged 16-44 years had had experience of anal intercourse in the year 2000 in the UK)
- forms of contraception and whether she has insisted on the use of a condom with a new partner despite having no need for contraception (if she has had a hysterectomy or is post-menopausal or he has had a vasectomy)
- her obstetric history and whether her children are still living at home
- gynaecological and especially menstrual history
- past sexual history.

In taking a sexual history, the medical history is important, especially to exclude diabetes, depression, heart and orthopaedic problems, hormone deficiencies, trauma and operations. Drugs taken, whether prescribed or recreational, alcohol intake and smoking habits should also be investigated.

Agreeing a management plan

After taking a history, the doctor or nurse will usually examine the patient, and a plan of management should be explained to her. Once you have her approval of what is to come, the rest should be much easier for both you and the patient. You will find that she will cooperate much better if she understands what you are trying to do, particularly with any medication.

Conclusion

A good history, carefully taken, will give the diagnosis in the majority of problems and can save a lot of repetitious questioning and missed diagnoses, while enabling the patient to be more comfortable in your presence.

Further reading

BBC. *Body language/communications skills.* www.bbc.co.uk/dna/ww2/A2431540 (last accessed 9 September 2004).

Godson S. *The sex book.* London: Cassell, 2003.

Gott M, Hinchliff S, Galena E. General practitioner attitudes to discussing sexual health issues with older people. *Soc Sci Med* 2004; **58**: 2093–103.

Guyatt GH, Haynes RB, Jaeschke RZ, *et al.* Users' guides to the medical literature: XXV. Evidence-based medicine: principles for applying the users' guides to patient care. Evidence-Based Medicine Working Group. *JAMA* 2000; **284**: 1290–6.

Johnson AM, Mercer CH, Erens B, *et al.* Sexual behaviour in Britain: partnerships, practices and HIV risk behaviours. *Lancet* 2000; **358**: 1835–42.

Morris D. *Man watching.* London: Triad Granada, 1980.

Tomlinson JM. Taking a sexual history. In, Tomlinson JM, ed. *ABC of sexual health.* Oxford: Blackwell/BMJ Books, 2005.

5 Psychosexual therapy and self-help

Rose Whiteley

Introduction
Psychosexual therapy
Self-help
Conclusion

Introduction

Sexual problems can be very isolating. Some people suffer in silence for years without discussing their concerns with anyone, perhaps even their sexual partners. Problems with sexual functioning can make us feel embarrassed, ashamed and stupid.

Fortunately, increasing numbers of professionals are specially trained to deal with sexual dysfunction: psychosexual therapists. Usually, their original training will have been in one of the psychological therapies or in medicine, but in addition they will have undertaken specialized training in:

- what makes for good sexual relationships
- the many causes of sexual dysfunction
- the range of therapies available – from physical treatments (for example, oral treatments, low-dose vaginal oestrogens or vacuum pumps) to talking treatments.

Psychosexual therapy (also referred to as sex therapy or psychosexual counselling) has been around since the 1950s and has proven success rates. Sex therapists regularly receive referrals from counsellors, psychotherapists, family doctors, hospital consultants, genitourinary medicine clinics and other medical professionals, and most will accept self-referrals.

Some patients, however, may be unable or unwilling to work on their problems with the help of a sex therapist – either through embarrassment or lack of time or resources; others may be sufficiently motivated to make use of self-help materials as an adjunct to individual or couples therapy.

Psychosexual therapy

For whom is sex therapy suitable?

Sex therapy is open to adults of all ages – lesbian, gay, bisexual or straight; married or unmarried; people with disabilities and the non-disabled; those living with chronic or terminal illness and those who are otherwise healthy.

Patients in an existing relationship generally are encouraged to attend sex therapy together. This is because sexual and relationship difficulties rarely (if ever) 'belong' to one partner or the other; the sexual problem will be having an impact on the way the couple relates, and the couple's behaviour will often perpetuate or intensify the original problem. Nevertheless, patients who do not have a sexual partner, or whose partner is not willing to attend, may often still find it helpful to attend sex therapy sessions on their own.

What kinds of problems can sex therapy help with?

Sex therapists can assess and treat the whole gamut of sexual dysfunctions, regardless of whether the main cause is physical, psychological or relational (Box 5.1). Non-medical sex therapists will refer patients for adjunctive medical treatments (such as phosphodiesterase type 5 inhibitors or hormone therapy) where organic factors are involved, if these are appropriate and the patient consents.

Types of presenting problems in psychosexual therapy include:

- loss of desire, in women and men
- difficulties with arousal – loss of sensation and insufficient lubrication for women and erectile dysfunction for men
- premature ejaculation
- dyspareunia – in women and men
- vaginismus
- anorgasmia (difficulty reaching orgasm) and retarded or absent ejaculation
- phobias, paraphilias and hypersexuality.

Box 5.1

Formulating the problem

After a detailed assessment, the therapist will be able to make an initial formulation of the problem by considering the convergence of physiological, psychological and relational aetiology in the context of the predisposing, precipitating and perpetuating factors involved. In sex therapy, however, treatment frequently serves a strong diagnostic function, and the diagnosis therefore will be kept under review as the effects of treatment are observed.

A paraphilia is an abnormal sexual behaviour, sexual anomaly or sexual deviation that is socially prohibited.

What does sex therapy involve?

Sex therapists are trained to be both knowledgeable and comfortable with talking about sex, and first and foremost, she or he will offer a safe and supportive space to find out what is going wrong and to discuss possible solutions.

The first few sessions involve taking a detailed social, medical, psychological, relationship and sexual history and finding out how the sexual problem is affecting the individuals concerned and their relationship. Following this, the therapist will give the couple information about how sexual problems arise and the various treatment options available, so that informed consent can be obtained (see Boxes 5.2, 5.3). They will be informed that homework tasks are likely to be assigned to facilitate and maintain changes and will be assured that all intimate work will take place in the privacy of their own home and never in the consulting room.

Box 5.2

Couples can unwittingly exacerbate their sexual problems: Case 1

A menopausal woman begins to find penetrative sex painful because her natural lubrication is slower to commence and less copious; no one has suggested she use an artificial lubricant. In response, her husband begins to 'get it over with quickly' so as not to prolong her discomfort, meaning she never reaches orgasm. As time goes on, she finds sex less and less physically and emotionally satisfying and her levels of arousal diminish further. In response, he gets faster and may even develop his own sexual dysfunctions – erectile dysfunction and/or premature ejaculation.

Box 5.3

Couples can unwittingly exacerbate their sexual problems: Case 2

A diabetic man in his 50s starts to experience erectile failure; he can generally get an erection but often loses it before penetration is possible. His partner, in an effort to be helpful, does everything she can not to 'distract' him from his erection, and they get into the habit of attempting intercourse the minute his erection is firm enough. Thus, their whole focus of attention is on getting and maintaining the erection, instead of on sharing a pleasant and intimate time and enjoying each other's bodies. As a result, his anxiety levels soar each time he manages to gain an erection, making failure inevitable; and she begins to feel resentful because none of her sexual needs are being met.

Psychosexual therapy involves an eclectic or integrated programme that draws on a number of different kinds of working. For instance, interventions might be psychoeducational (focusing on knowledge deficits), cognitive behavioural (focusing on patterns of thinking and behaviour that are causing difficulties), psychodynamic (which has more of an emphasis on the unconscious and exploring connections between the present and past events, especially developmental issues, than other types of therapy), humanistic (with an emphasis on personal responsibility and authenticity) or systemic (looking at the couple in context and finding out what is keeping the problem going). Examples of the kinds of interventions used include:

- sex education aimed at addressing knowledge deficits and dealing with unhelpful sexual myths, perhaps using books or videos
- exploration of the overall context for the sexual relationship, which may lead on to communication and conflict skills training or practical help with prioritization and work–life balance
- a 'personal sexual growth programme' to help each individual become more familiar and comfortable with his or her body and sexual self
- sensate focus, which involves a programme of sensual touching exercises concurrent with a ban on intercourse, so that physical intimacy and trust increase while performance anxiety subsides. The feedback in session from this task can be particularly helpful in providing additional diagnostic clues; for example, an unwillingness to carry out the genital touching phase can uncover a deeply held fear or shame or even a history of past sexual trauma
- specific behavioural exercises linked to particular problems, such as Kegel's exercises to strengthen pelvic muscles, the 'stop–start' technique to treat rapid ejaculation and a programme of relaxation and systematic desensitization for vaginismus
- conceptual frameworks, such as the Gestalt cycle of awareness (based on the idea that in life, we experience a continual cycle of emerging needs that may either be met or blocked in one way or another) in order to help clients identify their barriers to arousal and healthy sexual functioning
- examination of the therapeutic relationship and the dynamics in the room, which can help to uncover hidden conflicts or emotional wounds and facilitate healing.

How can patients obtain sex therapy?

The routes will vary between different countries. In the UK, the two main routes are through the National Health Service (NHS) or privately, depending on whether the couple is able and willing to pay. There may be a lengthy waiting list for NHS treatment but it will be free (although patients will have to pay privately for any prescriptions unless they are exempt). Private treatment generally will cost between £30 and £50 (€43–72; US$55–91) per session, but reduced fees sometimes are available, and patients are likely to be seen quickly and to have more choice about who they see.

Services vary widely across the UK, but depending on where patients live, sex therapy services may be available from the local family planning clinic, a genitourinary medicine clinic or a psychosexual unit within a larger hospital.

Psychosexual therapists should have specific qualifications in sex therapy and abide by the codes of ethics of an appropriate professional body.

Self-help

Nowadays, particularly since the Internet has become so popular, sexual materials of all kinds are easier than ever to find, and some of these have a useful role to play in enhancing our sensual and sexual lives.

The remainder of this chapter considers sexual products available in two areas: educational materials and those designed to enhance sexual arousal.

Self-education

A number of excellent books are available that can help women and men explore their sexual pleasures and difficulties. Many of these address common sexual assumptions and myths. Others take readers through a structured programme of exercises, offering very practical advice on overcoming problems. In addition, a number of helpful videos and DVDs are available, addressing both personal sexual growth and couple's issues.

Enhancing arousal

As discussed elsewhere, peri- and post-menopausal women often need more stimulation to become aroused and reach orgasm than they did before the menopause. A vast range of products are now readily available, and some women find these helpful to build excitement and facilitate a good sexual experience.

- **Vibrators:** Several new types of vibrators that resemble massagers or even objets d'art more than the traditional phalluses are available, although they do tend to be more expensive.

- **Clitoral stimulators:** Some are worn on the finger and do not need a battery; they can be used by the woman for self-pleasuring or on her by her partner.

- **Lubricants:** Many different water-based brands are now available, most of which resemble natural lubrication. Oil-based lubricants, such as peach kernel or sweet almond oils, which last longer than water-based lubricants, can be used, but they have the potential to break down the latex in condoms. This is important not only for contraception but for the prevention of sexually transmitted diseases.

- **Games:** Erotic board, dice or card games.
- **Lingerie** and fantasy 'dressing-up' clothes.

For years, 'erotica' often has been difficult to distinguish from pornography, as it largely has been confined to 'top-shelf' magazines aimed conspicuously at men. Nowadays, however, women who are comfortable with erotica are likely to find it increasingly easy to access – whether in print, on video or DVD or through websites containing sexual images and fiction.

Conclusion

Health professionals sometimes worry that if they 'open the floodgates' on a sexual difficulty they will soon find themselves out of their depth. There are, however, a wide range of professional and self-help resources that can be called on to assist with treating sexual problems.

Further reading

Berman J, Berman, L. *For women only. A revolutionary guide to reclaiming your sex life.* London: Virago Press, 2001.

Butcher J. A psychosexual approach to managing dyspareunia. *Practitioner* 2003; **247:** 484–9, 493–5.

Dickson A. *The mirror within: a new look at sexuality.* London: Quartet Books, 1985.

Godson S. *The sex book.* London: Cassel, 2002.

Johnston SL, Farrell SA, Bouchard C, *et al.* The detection and management of vaginal atrophy. *J Obstet Gynaecol Can* 2004; **26:** 503–15.

Kalamis C. *Women without sex: the truth about female sexual problems.* London: Self-Help Direct Publishing, 2003.

Kring B. Psychotherapy of sexual dysfunction. *Am J Psychother* 2000; **54:** 97–101.

Leiblum SR, Rosen RC, eds. *Principles and practice of sex therapy.* New York: Guilford Press, 2000.

Melnick J, Nevis S. Diagnosing in the here and now: a Gestalt therapy approach. In: Greenberg L, Watson J, Lietaer G, eds. *Handbook of experiential psychotherapy.* New York: Guilford Press, 1998: 428–65.

McGuire H, Hawton K. Interventions for vaginismus. *Cochrane Database Syst Rev* 2003; (1): CD001760.

Mosher DL. The Gestalt awareness-expression cycle as a model for sex therapy. *J Sex Marital Ther* 1977; **3:** 229–42.

Roos S. *Chronic sorrow.* New York: Brunner-Routledge, 2002.

Tomlinson JM, ed. *ABC of sexual health.* Oxford: Blackwell/BMJ Books, 2005.

Weeks GR, Gambescia N. *Erectile dysfunction: integrating couple therapy, sex therapy, and medical treatment.* New York: WW Norton, 2000.

Woldt A, Stein S. Gestalt therapy with the elderly: on 'coming of age' and 'completing Gestalts.' *Gestalt Review* 1997; **2**: 163–84.

Zilbergeld B. *A new male sexuality.* New York: Bantam Doubleday Dell Publishing, 1999.

6 Pharmacotherapy

Kevan Wylie

Introduction
Normal physiology of sex steroids
Androgen replacement therapy
Non-testosterone-based treatments
Conclusion

Introduction

Although increasingly criticized, the data from the National Health and Social Life Survey undertaken by Laumann *et al* (1999) provides evidence of a prevalence of sexual dysfunction in American women of around one-third of those sampled. One of the most common conditions is hypoactive sexual desire disorder (HSDD) (see Chapter 2); this is commonly referred to as a loss or lack of sexual desire or libido.

A lack of sexual desire is associated with a reduction or absence of sexual fantasies and/or sexual dreams. There may be somatic symptoms such as increased fatigability, tiredness, weakness and lack of energy, and there may be concurrent depressed mood. Other symptoms can include loss of muscle bulk and muscle weakness. The level of free testosterone level correlates significantly with both decreased desire and coital frequency in pre-menopausal women; so most therapy has been targeted towards androgen replacement.

Normal physiology of sex steroids

Oestrogen and androgen receptors have been found in the brain, with high concentrations of androgen receptors in the hypothalamus, pre-optic area hippocampus and other sites.

In women, slightly more than two-thirds of circulating testosterone is bound to sex hormone-binding globulin (SHBG), which is higher than the amount bound in men. A further third is weakly bound to albumin, which leaves around 2% of the total testosterone in the free or unbound state. As SHBG concentrations can fluctuate – for example, they are reduced in patients with clinical depression, in those taking corticosteroids and in women who have obesity, hypothyroidism or Cushing's syndrome (or androgen excess such as polycystic ovary syndrome). Sex hormone-binding globulin is raised in women who take exogenous oestrogens, women who are pregnant, women who have hyperthyroidism or cirrhosis, as well as with increasing age. Total testosterone, although the most common measure in clinical studies, does not yield meaningful information about tissue androgen exposure, as variations in SHBG levels in women can have dramatic effects on free testosterone levels. A free testosterone index accurately evaluates the tissue androgen status. Although the use of equilibrium dialysis would be the preferred choice for measuring free testosterone levels, many laboratories do not have this facility.

The recent attempt to measure serum androgen levels in pre-menopausal women with no complaints of sexual dysfunction established an age-related decrease in testosterone, free testosterone and the adrenal precursor dehydroepiandrosterone sulphate (DHEA-S). The free androgen index mirrored these decreases, confirming its usefulness in clinical practice. Sex hormone-binding globulin did not change throughout the pre-menopausal years. In 2004, Guay *et al* noted that pre-menopausal women with complaints of sexual dysfunction did, however, have lower levels of adrenal androgen precursors and testosterone than age-matched control women without such complaints. Further study is required to determine how low levels of adrenal androgens contribute to female sexual dysfunction.

During the natural menopause, a gradual decline of oestrogen levels occurs, as well as a temporary rise of serum testosterone levels secondary to the ovarian stromal hyperplasia, which lasts for up to five years. In women, the ovaries remain the primary site of production of testosterone, which is hydroxylated to dihydrotestosterone. Testosterone can also be aromatized to oestradiol. Precursor oestrogen hormones, such as androstenedione and DHEA, are produced in both the ovaries and the adrenals and both possess a less potent androgenic effect than testosterone. By the time women reach the age of 40 years, the mean circulating levels of testosterone are approximately half those of women in their twenties (Davis and Tran, 2001). In addition, DHEA and the sulphate product (DHEA-S) also decrease with age. Factors that affect ovarian production of these hormones include bilateral oophorectomy and use of gonadotrophin-releasing hormone (GnRH) analogues; some treatments for tumours can also reduce testosterone. An audit undertaken in the UK of 1170 consecutive hysterectomies found that in 630 cases, bilateral oophorectomy was undertaken at the same time. This was performed in 22% of hysterectomies undertaken in women aged under 40 years and 54% in those aged 40–49 years. Testosterone can also be reduced by any factors that increase the levels of SHBG, such as oestrogen therapy in oral contraceptives. Accurate measurement of both testosterone and androstenedione is essential and is usually undertaken in the early morning in the middle third of the menstrual cycle.

Androgen replacement therapy

Androgen replacement therapy is indicated following both natural and surgical menopause, in women taking treatments that bring about ovarian failure and in those taking oestrogenic steroid therapy.

Testosterone

Several studies to date have shown a benefit of testosterone therapy in post-menopausal women. In women with surgically induced menopause, Shifren *et al* (2000) reported increased sexual activity, greater frequency of intercourse and greater frequency and quality of orgasms, as well as an improvement of the brief index of sexual functioning for women (BISF) rating scale, in women using testosterone patches. In total, five randomized, double-blind, controlled trials have evaluated testosterone supplementation either alone or in combination with oestrogen, with three of the five studies showing significant benefit (Miller, 2003).

In the UK, the only licensed preparation for post-menopausal replacement of testosterone is subcutaneous implants. These are usually implanted at the same time as oestrogen replacement. Pellets of 50 mg can be inserted and will usually show effect for four to six months. Side-effects are rare but include fluid retention and a decrease in high-density lipoprotein cholesterol. There seems to be no increase in risk in either breast cancer or endometrial hyperplasia by the addition of androgen therapy. Sources of androgen currently available for men, including intramuscular injection and transdermal gels, can be used in women in smaller doses. Alternative preparations for testosterone under investigation include transdermal patches. A recent study of 562 surgically menopausal women with HSDD who received a testosterone transdermal patch found a 74% increase in the frequency of total satisfaction with sexual activity, as well as a 56% increase in sexual desire compared with baseline.

Testosterone therapy has also been noted to result in an increase in vasocongestion within the vagina in response to erotic visual stimulation in women with hypothalamic amenorrhoea.

Dehydroepiandrosterone

Dehydroepiandrosterone (DHEA) and DHEA-S, the androgen precursors made in the adrenal glands, are converted to testosterone. Only one double-blind, placebo-controlled, crossover study of DHEA over a four month period has been done, and this was in women with adrenal insufficiency and low DHEA. The study found that DHEA improved well-being and sexuality. Side-effects of DHEA include a decrease in high-density lipoprotein and total cholesterol.

Tibolone
Tibolone is a steroid agent that has tissue specific oestrogenic, androgenic and progestogenic actions. It is converted to three metabolites: two have oestrogenic properties on the vagina, bone and menopausal symptoms and the third is formed in the endometrium, with progestrogenic and androgenic activity. In post-menopausal woman, tibolone has a positive effect on the vagina, mood, menopausal symptoms, bone and sexual well-being but without stimulation of the breast or endometrium. A number of studies have found tibolone to enhance sexual function, as well as to significantly increase vaginal blood flow in response to erotic fantasy.

Non-testosterone-based treatments

Vaginal oestrogens

Low-dose vaginal oestrogens are effective treatments for vaginal dryness and dyspareunia. Synthetic oestrogens should be avoided, as they are well absorbed from the vagina. The options available are low-dose natural oestrogens, such as vaginal oestriol by cream or pessary or oestradiol by tablet or ring. Long-term treatment is required, as symptoms return on cessation of therapy. With the recommended dose regimens, no adverse endometrial effects occur, and a progestogen need not be added for endometrial protection with such low-dose preparations.

Sildenafil

Sildenafil is the first selective inhibitor of phosphodiesterase 5 (PDE-5) and is mainly used in erectile dysfunction (see Chapter 10). Data for its use in post-menopausal women are limited. Trials have evaluated the use of sildenafil in women with female sexual arousal disorder (FSAD). Results are conflicting and further data are awaited.

Bupropion

Bupropion is an antidepressant that inhibits reuptake of noradrenaline and dopamine. It is mainly used for smoking cessation; however, it may also improve sexual function. A double-blind, placebo-controlled study for 12 weeks in 51 women found that bupropion, titrated up to a maximum of

450 mg/day, led to a greater increase in ratings for sex drive, with similar results seen in a single-blind, placebo-controlled study. It may also be an effective antidote to elective serotonin reuptake inhibitor-induced sexual dysfunction. Further data are awaited.

Conclusion

Several therapeutic options are available for a naturally occurring change in the hormonal milieu of menopausal women who complain of sexual symptoms and seek treatment. Attention to other aspects of relationship issues is crucial, and complete reliance on endocrinological and pharmacological treatments is likely to result in poor outcomes.

Further reading

Arlt W, Callies F, van Vlijmen JC, *et al*. Dehydroepiandrosterone replacement in women with adrenal insufficiency. *N Engl J Med* 1999; **341**: 1013–20.

Bachmann G, Bancroft J, Braunstein G, *et al*. Female androgen insufficiency: the Princeton consensus statement on definition, classification, and assessment. *Fertil Steril* 2002; **77**: 660–5.

Basson R, McInnes R, Smith MD, *et al*. Efficacy and safety of sildenafil in estrogenized women with sexual dysfunction associated with female sexual arousal disorder. *Obstet Gynecol* 2000; **95**: S1–54.

Berman JR, Berman LA, Toler SM, *et al*. Safety and efficacy of sildenafil citrate for the treatment of female sexual arousal disorder: a double-blind, placebo controlled study. *J Urol* 2003; **170**: 2333–8.

Cameron DR, Braunstein GD. Androgen replacement therapy in women. *Fertil Steril* 2004; **82**: 273–89.

Clayton AH, Warnock JK, Kornstein SG, *et al*. A placebo-controlled trial of bupropion SR as an antidote for selective serotonin reuptake inhibitor-induced sexual dysfunction. *J Clin Psychiatry* 2004; **65**: 62–7.

Davis S. Testosterone and sexual desire in women. *J Sex Educ Ther* 2000: **25**: 25–32.

Davis SR. The use of testosterone after menopause. *J Br Menopause Soc* 2004; 10: 65–9.

Davis S, Tran J. What are 'normal' testosterone levels for women? *J Clin Endocrinol Metab* 2001; **86**: 1842–4.

Guay A, Munarriz R, Jacobson J, *et al*. Serum androgen levels in healthy premenopausal women with and without sexual dysfunction: Part A. Serum androgen levels in women aged 20–49 years with no complaints of sexual dysfunction. *Int J Impot Res* 2004: **16**: 112–20.

Guay A, Jacobson J, Munarriz R, *et al*. Serum androgen levels in healthy premenopausal women with and without sexual dysfunction: Part B: Reduced serum androgen levels in healthy premenopausal women with complaints of sexual dysfunction. *Int J Impot Res* 2004; **16**: 121–9.

Kaplan SA, Reis RB, Kohn IJ, *et al*. Safety and efficacy of sildenafil in postmenopausal women with sexual dysfunction. *Urology* 1999; **53**: 481–6.

Laan E, Van Lunsenrhw RH, Everard W. The effects of tibolone on vaginal blood flow, sexual desire and arousability in postmenopausal women. *Climacteric* 2001; **4**: 28–41.

Laumann E O, Paik A, Rosen RC. Sexual dysfunction in the United States: prevalence and predictors. *JAMA* 1991; **281**: 537–44.

Mackenzie IZ, Naish C, Rees M, Manek S. 1170 hysterectomies: indications and pathology. *J Br Menopause Soc* 2004; **10**: 108–12.

Miller HB, Hunt JS. Female sexual dysfunction: review of the disorder and evidence for available treatment alternatives. *J Pharm Pract* 2003; **16**: 200–8.

Modell JG, May RS, Katholi CR. Effect of bupropion-SR on orgasmic dysfunction in non-depressed subjects: a pilot study. *J Sex Marit Ther* 2000; **26**: 231–40.

Modelska K, Cummings S. Female sexual dysfunction in postmenopausal women: systematic review of placebo-controlled trials. *Am J Obstet Gynecol* 2003; **188**: 286–93.

Nathorst-Böös J, Hammar M. Effect on sexual life – a comparison between tibolone and a continuous estradiol-norethisterone acetate regimen. *Maturitas* 1997: **26**: 15–20.

Segraves R T, Croft H, Kavoussi R, *et al.* Bupropion sustained release (SR) for the treatment of hypoactive sexual desire disorder (HSDD) in non-depressed women. *J Sex Marit Ther* 2001; **27**: 303–16.

Shifren JL, Braunstein GD, Simon JA, *et al.* Transdermal testosterone treatment in women with impaired sexual function after oophorectomy. *N Engl J Med* 2000; **343**: 682–8.

Suckling J, Lethaby A, Kennedy R. Local oestrogen for vaginal atrophy in postmenopausal women. *Cochrane Database Syst Rev* 2003; (4): CD001500.

Wu M-H, Pan S-T W, Hsu C-C, *et al.* Quality of life and sexuality changes in postmenopausal women receiving tibolone therapy. *Climacteric* 2001; **4**: 314–19.

7 Contraception in the peri-menopause

Ailsa Gebbie

Introduction
Fertility and pregnancy in older women
Methods of contraception
Hormone replacement therapy
Conclusion

Introduction

The peri-menopause is a time of life when declining ovarian function causes menstrual dysfunction and the onset of menopausal symptoms. Although fertility is low, it is not zero, and a late unplanned pregnancy can have devastating consequences. Women may have anxieties about using particular methods at that particular time, and many abandon contraception altogether before they become menopausal. Clinicians need to be able to give clear advice about which methods of contraception are suitable and when contraception can be discontinued.

Fertility and pregnancy in older women

Oocyte quality is undoubtedly the main factor in age-related fertility decline. In the mid-to-late thirties, there is acceleration in spontaneous follicle atresia from the ovaries, and oocytes are more susceptible to aneuploidy (an abnormality of chromosome number that is not an exact multiple of the haploid number) and mitochondrial mutations.

Pregnancies in women aged over 50 years are rare. The oldest known woman to give birth following a spontaneous conception was 57 years and 129 days. Assisted conception techniques have made pregnancies possible well into the post-menopausal age range but only by using donor eggs.

Women aged over 40 years have a higher abortion rate per total pregnancy rate than any other age group, and in the UK, more than 40% of all pregnancies in this age group will end in therapeutic abortion. Older women also have increased rates of miscarriage – due principally to chromosomal abnormalities – and are more likely to have a child with Down's syndrome.

They also have a higher risk of pregnancy-induced hypertension and gestational diabetes.

Methods of contraception

In the Western world, where contraceptive choice is available, striking changes have been seen in patterns of contraceptive use with age. For example, while use of oral contraception peaks to nearly 60% in the twenties, less than 20% of women are using this form of contraception over the age of 40 years.

Combined oral contraception

There is no upper age limit for use of combined oral contraception (COC) by healthy, low risk, non-smoking women, who in practice may continue with it until the age of around 50 years. Women who smoke must always be advised to discontinue COC use at the age of 35 years. Although COC has small risks, there is a significant package of non-contraceptive benefits, which may be particularly appropriate for an individual older woman. In 1996 the World Health Organization stated that for women aged 40 years and over the advantages of using the oral contraceptive pill generally outweigh any theoretical or proven risks.

Cardiovascular disease
The incidence of arterial disease with COC is now extremely small, as low-dose pills are universally prescribed, and women with significant risk factors for arterial disease rarely take them. At any given age, a woman who uses COC and smokes is at a greater risk of death from arterial disease than a user of COC who does not. The annual risk of death from cardiovascular disease attributable to COC use is 20–25 per million users aged 40–44 years, which is up to 10 times greater than among those aged 20–24 years.

Venous thromboembolism
Venous thromboembolism (VTE) is the most common cardiovascular event among users of COC. The associated mortality is relatively low compared with that associated with arterial diseases. It is well established that COC use increases the risk of venous thromboembolism at least 3–6 fold, and the risk seems highest in the first year of use. Although risk of VTE increases with age, older COC users do not seem to have an increased relative risk compared with younger users.

Cancer
The potential relationship between COC use and various cancers is summarized in Table 7.1.

Table 7.1

Summary of relationship between combined oral contraception and various cancers.

Cancer	Potential effect of COC (RR)
Breast	1.24 in current and recent users
Cervical	2.2 after 10 years' use
Endometrial	0.5 after 5 years' use
Ovarian	0.3 after 12 years' use
Colorectal	0.6 after 7 years' use

RR, recurrence rate; COC, combined oral contraception

The added risk of breast cancer among current COC users takes 10 years to return to normal after stopping therapy. Among 10,000 women aged 40–44 years who used COC for five years, 262 cases of breast cancer would be expected up to the age of 55 years – 32 more cases than among never users (230 cases per 10,000 women). Although long duration use of COC seems to be associated with an increased risk of cervical cancer, it is simply not known whether there is any lasting effect at older ages after COC use has ceased. The risks of endometrial, ovarian and colorectal cancer are all reduced with long-term COC use. It also reduces the incidence of benign breast disease, particularly development of fibroadenomas and cystic disease, and decreases the risk of functional ovarian cysts.

Menstrual benefits
Peri-menopausal women frequently experience heavy, painful, irregular menstruation. Combined oral contraception controls menstrual blood loss, reducing it by around 44%. Users of COCs have significantly fewer hospital referrals for menstrual problems and avoid hysterectomy.

Osteoporosis
Evidence-based analysis suggests that COC has a favourable effect on bone mineral density. Long-term users seem to reach the menopause with bone density 2–3% higher than non-users, but it is not known whether this effect confers any benefit to prevent lifetime fracture.

Progestogen-only methods

All progestogen-only methods can be associated with both menstrual irregularity and amenorrhoea. They can be prescribed for older women with contraindications to COC, in particular women aged over 35 years who smoke or have other risk factors for cardiovascular disease. There seems to be no significant increase in the relative risk of stroke, myocardial infarction or venous thromboembolic disease among women using progestogen-only methods.

Progestogen-only pills (POP)

Although the overall failure rate of the progestogen-only pill (POP) is 2–3 per hundred women-years (HWY), among women aged over 40 years, it is only 0.3 per HWY because of increased inhibition of ovulation at older ages.

A desogestrel-containing POP, associated with significant inhibition of ovulation compared to standard POP preparations, is now available. There seem to be no particular advantages in using it in peri-menopausal women, who are of low fertility, compared with standard POP preparations.

Depot medroxyprogesterone acetate

The intramuscular injection of 150 mg depot medroxyprogesterone acetate (DMPA) is an extremely effective contraceptive method for women of all ages. It will help dysmenorrhoea and menorrhagia and is a useful strategy to treat premenstrual syndrome. It has few side-effects and most long-term users will become amenorrhoeic. Because DMPA has significantly suppressive effects on ovarian production of oestradiol, concerns about its prolonged use and development of osteoporosis remain. At present, it is not possible to give a definitive evidence-based answer. Some data are very reassuring and show similar bone density in past users of DMPA and those who have never used it. Other data suggest that any bone loss is transient and reversible following cessation of therapy. There is no consensus on whether it is of value to check an oestradiol level, perform a 'routine' bone density scan or prescribe exogenous oestrogen to long-term or older DMPA users.

It is probably prudent to consider discontinuing DMPA at around the age of 45 years in most women to allow for any spontaneous recovery of bone density prior to the actual menopause. For some women, the menstrual advantages of using DMPA far outweigh any theoretical risk of developing osteoporosis.

Etonorgestrel implant

Implanon is a single polyethylene vinyl acetate rod inserted subdermally into the upper arm; it releases the progestogen etonorgestrel at a dose of around 67 mg/day. It is effective for up to three years and is generally well tolerated, with 82% of women in clinical trials continuing its use beyond two years. Most of the research studies on the implant excluded women aged over 40 years, but there is no reason that would contraindicate its use in women purely because of age.

Hormonal emergency contraception

In the UK, levonorgestrel-only has become the hormonal emergency contraception of choice, has virtually no contraindications and is now available for purchase over the counter without prescription. Levonorgestrel emergency contraception can be recommended for a woman of any age if an episode of unprotected intercourse has occurred and she is deemed to be at risk of pregnancy. It is effective if the dose is taken within 72 hours of unprotected intercourse and should be taken as a single dose (1500 µg) as soon as possible.

Intra-uterine device (IUD)

The modern copper IUD is a highly effective and cost effective method of contraception for women of all ages. Older women who use IUDs have a lower incidence of pelvic infection, expulsion and failure, including ectopic pregnancy, compared with younger IUD users. The majority of all women who use IUDs have a modest increase in menstrual blood loss and a degree of increased dysmenorrhoea. Peri-menopausal women with an IUD *in situ* may well experience bleeding difficulties, although this menstrual disturbance is generally related to hormonal factors and their effect on the endometrium rather than the device itself. It is standard practice that a copper IUD inserted after the age of 40 years can remain in place, without being changed until the user becomes menopausal.

Intrauterine system (IUS)

The intrauterine system (IUS), which releases 20 µg levonorgestrel per day, has particular advantages for peri-menopausal woman in terms of highly effective contraception and control of menstrual dysfunction, reducing menstrual blood loss by around 90%.

The IUS is licensed for use as the progestogen component of hormone replacement therapy (HRT) in many countries. The combination of systemic oestrogen and an IUS has been shown to diminish menopausal symptoms and induce endometrial atrophy. The probability of irregular bleeding and spotting in the first few months after insertion is high, although thereafter amenorrhoea is common. Some difficulty in inserting the existing IUS may be encountered in some older women, and a low-dose smaller IUS is in development.

Barrier methods

Most contraceptive surveys show steady use of condoms across the age ranges. Sexually transmitted infections are not respecters of age, and older individuals entering into new relationships must be advised to consider personal protection against infection (see Chapter 8). The diaphragm is a low-risk, woman-controlled method of contraception that older women use more reliably, with significantly lower failure rates, than younger users.

Sterilization

The sterilization rates for both men and women in the UK are significantly higher than in many other European countries. Around 45% of peri-menopausal women rely on a permanent surgical procedure for contraception; this contrasts with France, where the figure is only around 11%. Common sense dictates that peri-menopausal women, who are very close to natural sterility, should avoid a surgical procedure, but women should be assessed individually. Women who are sterilized at older ages are much less likely to regret having the procedure performed.

Stopping contraception

The general advice about stopping contraception is that women should continue contraception for one year following their last spontaneous menstrual period if aged over 50 years. Women under the age of 50 should continue with contraception for two further years following their last period to exclude the likelihood of further ovulation. Levels of hormones, such as follicle-stimulating hormone (FSH), fluctuate widely during the peri-menopause, and, in general, it is not helpful to check hormone levels to give guidance on when contraception can be stopped.

Stopping the combined pill

It is good practice to advise most women to stop the combined pill at the age of 50 years, as around 50% will already be post-menopausal. Women who use COC for contraception can be advised to change to a progesterone-only pill if she prefers a hormonal method, or else a barrier method. This will allow assessment of her menstrual cycle, menopausal status and thereby her requirements for contraception or HRT.

Stopping the progestogen-only pill

Women aged over 50 years who are taking a POP and are amenorrhoeic can have a check of their serum FSH level; in contrast to COC users, this will give an accurate assessment of their underlying menopausal status. If FSH is elevated, the POP can be discontinued after one further year.

Hormone replacement therapy

Once a peri-menopausal woman has commenced hormone replacement therapy (HRT), it becomes impossible to assess accurately when natural sterility has been achieved. Conventional sequential HRT is not a reliable contraceptive, and women may still ovulate. Barrier methods of contraception – an IUD or the POP – can all be continued in conjunction with HRT. Although no scientific evidence confirms the efficacy of the POP in this respect, it is now often recommended, and logically it should be effective.

In practice, it usually is most convenient to recommend that women who started HRT when they were peri-menopausal should continue contraception up to the age of 55 years, when natural sterility can be assumed.

Conclusion

Peri-menopausal women have low fertility but a major requirement for highly effective contraception. All methods of contraception become more effective with age, and no method is contraindicated because of age alone. Future research should examine the interface between hormonal contraception and HRT, with a view to developing even safer, low-dose hormonal combinations that will allow women to surf through the peri-menopause with ease.

Further reading

Burkman R, Schlesselman JJ, Zieman M. Safety concerns and health benefits associated with oral contraception. *Am J Obstet Gynecol* 2004; **190 (4 Suppl)**: S5–22.

Drugs and Therapeutic Bulletin. Etonogestrel implant (Implanon) for contraception. *Drug Ther Bull* 2001; **39**: 57–9.

Faculty of Family Planning and Reproductive Health Care Clinical Effectiveness Unit. FFPRHC Guidance (April 2004). The levonorgestrel-releasing intrauterine system (LNG-IUS) in contraception and reproductive health. *J Fam Plann Reprod Health Care* 2004; **30**: 99–108.

Gallo MF, Grimes DA, Schulz KF. Cervical cap versus diaphragm for contraception. *Cochrane Database Syst Rev* 2002; **(4)**: CD003551.

Gebbie A. Contraception in the perimenopause. *J Br Menopause Soc* 2003; **9**: 123–8.

Guinness World Records. *Guinness book of records*. Guinness World Records Limited. London: Bantam Books, 2000.

Jick H, Kaye JA, Vasilakis-Scaramozza C, Jick S. Risk of venous thromboembolism among users of third generation oral contraceptives compared with users of oral contraceptives with levonorgestrel before and after 1995: cohort and case-control analysis. *BMJ* 2000; **321**: 1190–5.

Kunhong W, Borgatta L, Stubblefield P. Low dose oral contraceptives and bone mineral density: an evidence-based analysis. *Contraception* 2000; **61**: 77–82.

Larsson G, Milson I, Lindstedt G, Rybo G. The influence of low-dose combined oral contraception on menstrual blood loss and iron status. *Contraception* 1992; **46**: 327–34.

Orr-Walker BJ, Evans MC, Ames RW, *et al*. The effect of past use of the injectable contraceptive depot medroxyprogesterone acetate on bone mineral density in normal postmenopausal women. *Clin Endocrinol* 1998; **49**: 615–18.

Pal L, Santoro N. Age-related decline in fertility. *Endocrinol Metab Clin North Am* 2003; **32**: 669–88.

Practice Committee of the American Society for Reproductive Medicine. Hormonal contraception: Recent advances and controversies. *Fertil Steril* 2004; **82**: 520–6.

Trussell J, Ellertson C, Stewart F, *et al*. The role of emergency contraception. *Am J Obstet Gynecol* 2004; **190(4 Suppl)**: S30–8.

Vessey M, Painter R, Mant J. Oral contraception and other factors in relation to hospital referral for menstrual problems without known underlying cause: findings in a large cohort study. *Br J Fam Plann* 1996; **22**: 166–9.

Vessey MP, Lawless M, Yeats D, McPherson K. Progestogen only oral contraception. Findings in a large prospective study with special reference to effectiveness. *Br J Fam Plann* 1985; **10**: 117–21.

Westhoff C. Bone mineral density and DMPA. *J Reprod Med* 2002; **47** (**9 Suppl**): 795–9.

World Health Organization. *Improving access to quality care in Family Planning. Medical Eligibility Criteria for Contraceptive Use.* Geneva: World Health Organization, 1996. WHO/FRH/FPP/96.9.

World Health Organization. Cardiovascular disease and use of oral and injectable progestogen-only contraceptive and combined injectable contraceptives. Results of an international multicentre, case-control study. *Contraception* 1998; **57**: 315–24.

8 Sexually transmitted infections

Faryal Mahar and Jackie Sherrard

Introduction
Scale of the problem
Factors that predispose older people to STIs
Presentation of STIs
Symptom recognition
HIV and the menopause
Conclusion

Introduction

Traditionally, older people are not perceived to be at risk of sexually transmitted infections (STIs), but several factors may predispose them towards a higher infection rate. It is not possible to distinguish between sexually transmitted infections and other genital pathology from genital symptoms alone, and hence accurate diagnosis is required. In addition, post-menopausal women present with an array of symptoms that may be attributed to either the effect of lacking hormones or a sexually transmitted infection. The differential gets even more complicated when women who have had a previous hysterectomy present with a mixture of symptoms.

Scale of the problem

Little international data exist on STI rates in older women, but according to the American Center for Disease Control (CDC) data, a consistently increasing number of older adults are being infected with sexually transmitted infections, particularly with HIV/AIDS (Table 8.1). The current American figures show that 18% of people with HIV infection with or without AIDS were aged over 45 years. The most rapidly growing group of patients are those who acquire infection through heterosexual contact. Heterosexual transmission as a risk in older adults increased from 6% of cases in 1992 to 13% by the end of 1997. Older adults have limited information about acquisition of STIs, including HIV/AIDS, compared with their younger counterparts. Although they are at a significant risk of acquiring a sexually

Table 8.1

Age at diagnosis of AIDS as of December 1998
(CDC, 1998)

Age (years)	Number (%)
Male	
40–49	152,154 (26.5)
>50	62,070 (10.8)
Female	
30–39	49,640 (41)
40–49	24,085 (21)
>50	10,091 (9)

CDC, Center for Disease Control

transmitted infection, they are almost universally omitted from prevention programmes.

Within the United Kingdom, data are available for women attending genitourinary (GUM) clinics, and in 2003, 2601 women aged 45 years and above were diagnosed with a range of STIs (Table 8.2). These figures, by their very nature, do not include older women managed for STIs outside

Table 8.2

Selected STIs seen in GUM clinics in 2003 in England, Wales and Northern Ireland, by age (Health Protection Agency, 2004)

Condition	Sex	Age group (years)		
		35–44	45–64	>64
Primary and secondary infectious syphilis	Male	474	227	14
	Female	27	15	1
Uncomplicated gonorrhoea	Male	2986	1082	53
	Female	548	138	2
Uncomplicated chlamydial infection	Male	4017	996	57
	Female	2052	412	24
Anogenital herpes simplex (first attack)	Male	1519	624	51
	Female	1518	739	18
Anogenital warts (first attack)	Male	5116	2075	151
	Female	2809	1196	56

of GUM clinics or women with other conditions where an age breakdown of diagnoses is not available. In the years between 1995 and 2003, some infections have shown marked increases in women aged 45 to 64 years, with infectious syphilis increasing by 275%, Chlamydia by 175% and gonorrhoea by 254%.

Factors that predispose older people to STIs

Changes in social norms with divorce and new partners

Older women are perceived to be relatively sexually inactive and assumed to be in a monogamous heterosexual relationship. This is a time in life when long-term relationships may have broken down and women are forming new sexual relationships, but as women in this age group are post-menopausal, sterilized or hysterectomized, the use of barrier methods of contraception is infrequent. Unprotected sexual intercourse thus puts them at a higher risk of acquiring an STI.

A national survey from 1990 to 1991 found that more than 2% of older Americans reported having two or more sexual partners in the preceding year. Average frequency of sexual activity of people aged 50 years or older has been estimated to be two to four times a month.

Male factors

Although reduced sexual activity is seen with increasing age, a substantial number of older men continue to be sexually active. Both health status and partner's responsiveness have been found to be moderators of the age effect, and in the absence of any health issues or social isolation, many men keep active sexual lifestyles.

In a study performed by Gott in 2001 on older community-based adults aged over 50 years, it was found that more than 80% were sexually active, while 7% engaged in risky sexual behaviours that placed them at risk of a sexually transmitted infection. Risk takers were typically male, aged between 50 and 60 years and married. Two-thirds previously had shown health concerns and had either presented to a GUM clinic or had seen their primary-care physician.

Older adults may be at a higher risk due to their age and the combination of denial and extreme secrecy. Risk taking may be compounded by an already compromized immune system related to age or other age-related health problems. Erectile dysfunction may render use of condoms difficult and hence impair their effectiveness. Older adults assume that they are safe because they are in a monogamous, or nearly monogamous, relationship and know their partners. They happen to be in a state of denial or near denial, with a strong belief that they are not at risk or that 'they are old'. Some may be reluctant to report risky behaviour due to stigmatization, marginalization and inadequate information provided to this age group.

The effect of oestrogen deficiency and risk of a sexually transmitted infection

Older women are at higher risk of STI acquisition because of physiological changes that occur naturally as part of the ageing process. With increasing age, there is a gradual decline of immune function and the presence of intercurrent disease, which may predispose individuals to acquisition of HIV and other STIs. Reduced vaginal secretions, thinning of the vaginal mucosa and increased friability of vaginal and cervical tissue due to oestrogen deficiency may result in tears and microabrasions that lead to increased susceptibility to STIs, particularly to HIV. This may be compounded by the fact that there is increased use of drugs by the partner for erectile dysfunction (see Chapter 10).

Oestrogen is thought to enhance the pathogenicity of many urogenital organisms and may lead to increased incidence of infection among post-menopausal women who receive hormone replacement therapy (HRT). Those using HRT may be more prone to vulvovaginal candidiasis, as oestrogen has been shown to enhance vaginal avidity for *Candida albicans* and to stimulate its transformation from the yeast form to pathogenic hyphae.

Trichomonas vaginalis has specific oestrogen receptors, which suggests a mechanism for increased susceptibility to trichomoniasis in users of HRT.

There are multiple risk factors for heterosexual transmission of HIV in women. In menopausal women, in particular, one of the factors may be thinning of the vaginal epithelium. The utilization of HRT, especially combined with progestogens, may compound vaginal epithelial thinning and predispose the mucosa to microabrasions and HIV transmission. A study of simian immunodeficiency virus (SIV) in macaques indicated that progesterone might be associated with increased risk of acquisition of SIV secondary to thinning of vaginal epithelium. Data from humans have shown that progesterone-dominant conditions and genital ulcer disease are associated with an increase in CC chemokine receptor 5 (CCR5) for HIV on cervical epithelium, providing another mechanism whereby hormonal manipulation may increase the risk of transmission.

HPV infection

Human papillomavirus (HPV) infections are highly prevalent, especially among young sexually active women. Although the great majority of HPV infections in women resolve within one year, they are a major concern because persistent infection with specific types (16, 18, 31, 33, 35 and 45) are causally related to cervical cancer. These types also cause cervical smear abnormalities. Other types (6 and 11) cause genital warts and low-grade cytological abnormalities.

Routine cervical screening has reduced the incidence of cervical cancer in the developed world; however, this is not the case in developing countries, where cervical cancer represents a major cause of death. Cervical cancer and HPV infection share the same risk factors, but while HPV infection is found in young women (aged <30 or 40 years), cervical cancer is seen in the fifth or sixth decades. The decline in the incidence of HPV infection seen after the age of approximately 40 years is consistent with immunological clearance of the organism, whereas the development of cervical cancer is associated with persistence of the virus.

Persistence of HPV infection is seen especially with underlying HIV infection, where the level of immune suppression is high. In HIV-negative women with cervical intraepithelial neoplasia (CIN) 2 and 3, the risk of recurrence or persistence of CIN 2 or 3 after one year of treatment is 5–10%, whereas the recurrence rate remains high in HIV-positive women. Palefsky and colleagues have also provided information that a low CD4 positive lymphocyte count and a high viral load (>100,000 copies/ml) are independent factors associated with HPV infection.

Presentation of STIs

Most STIs are commonly asymptomatic and the symptoms that occur are often due to local complications. Wart virus infection presents either as macroscopic genital warts or as an abnormality on cervical smear. Genital herpes simplex may present with vulval ulceration, but recurrent infection, in particular, may present as vulval soreness, superficial dyspareunia or dysuria.

Vaginal discharge, vaginitis, vulvitis and/or superficial dyspareunia may all be presentations of vaginal infection with trichomoniasis, bacterial vaginosis or candidiasis, and less commonly endocervical infection with Chlamydia or gonorrhoea. Gonorrhoea and Chlamydia are frequently asymptomatic but may present as pelvic pain, deep dyspareunia and menstrual disturbance, including intermenstrual and post-coital bleeding.

It will be noted that all these symptoms are non-specific and may be attributed to menopausal symptoms or more sinister pathology if an STI is not considered in the differential diagnosis.

Symptom recognition

There is a delay between symptom recognition and health care presentation (Gott, 1999). The level of delay shown by the older population is high, with

43.8% waiting for at least two weeks before presenting. This may imply that this age group is ill informed about genitourinary symptoms or may not perceive themselves to be at risk of infection. Many women suffer from other genital skin conditions such as vulvovaginal thrush, lichen sclerosis, vulval eczema/dermatitis or psoriasis. Self-treatment and waiting for symptoms to resolve could be a possible reason for delayed presentation. Other reasons in delayed presentation include: wanting to 'wait and see' whether symptoms improved or got worse, embarrassment and thinking 'symptoms were normal'.

HIV and the menopause

As the number of ageing people with HIV increases, the implications for disease progression are becoming clearer, with advancing age related to a shorter time of progression to AIDS and death. The effect of the menopause/older age on HIV disease progression is still unclear, but it may be related to the poor immune functional ability with advancing age.

Older adults (36%) are more likely to present with advanced HIV disease, including AIDS, compared with their younger counterparts (5%). In older adults, there is a lack of suspicion of HIV among both patients and clinicians, and there is a shorter and less symptomatic pre-AIDS phase. Clinical deterioration is more rapid among older HIV-infected people than among younger adults. The difference may be due to the fact that there is a more rapid loss of CD4 helper cells in older adults compared with younger people.

Comorbid conditions, such as heart disease, chronic pulmonary disease and diabetes, may be present, along with HIV-related opportunistic conditions. The presence of age-related illnesses may have a deleterious effect on the progression of AIDS and may contribute to rapid death. Response to therapy and the development of serious side effects to HIV drug therapy are all modified by age. A study by van Benthem found that post-menopausal women had lower CD4 lymphocyte counts three years after seroconversion than pre-menopausal women (333 versus 399×10^6 cells/l; p-value=0.09), suggesting that CD4 lymphocyte counts differ between pre-menopausal and post-menopausal women – perhaps because of changes in the level of reproductive hormones in the menopause.

Clinical presentation of older HIV patients does not differ from that of their younger counterparts; however, HIV may be misdiagnosed as the symptom presentation, such as fatigue, anorexia, weight loss, night sweats and memory problems, are non-specific and mimic symptoms of age-related disorders, including menopausal symptoms. Symptoms of recurrent vaginal thrush have been reported in 37% of women as one of the first presenting features of HIV infection. Bacterial pneumonia occurred in 13% of initial illness, while systemic symptoms such as fever, drenching sweats and weight loss occurred in 7% of women.

It can be challenging to distinguish between age-related conditions or menopause-related problems and HIV-related symptoms, or those associated with both. The differential diagnosis is complex, as many older adults may have multiple diagnoses. Bacterial infections, such as pneumonia, herpes virus infections, including herpes zoster, and other infections seen in older adults may be treated correctly without the suspicion of HIV infection as the causal factor. HIV dementia may present as altered mental status, impaired recent memory or decreased intellect and so may mimic Alzheimer's or Parkinson's disease.

Conclusion

In the current era of mass media messages about safer sexual practices and healthy lifestyle, it is important to include this generation of older people. As increased numbers of relationships break down and partnerships change, older people are potentially at risk of acquiring sexually transmitted infections with serious sequelae and may be unaware of the risks.

Menopausal women have largely been ignored within the field of sexual health. With the increased ageing population of the UK having a more liberal attitude towards sex, there is likely to be a continuing rise in STIs in this age group. Evidence suggests that menopausal women are a vulnerable group, and with the current dramatic rise in STIs in all age groups, it strongly suggests that clinicians caring for these individuals should be aware of the risk. Risk assessment and referral for screening for infections should be carried out where appropriate.

Further reading

Adler WH, Nagel JE. Acquired immunodeficiency syndrome in the elderly. *Drugs Aging* 1994; **4**: 410–16.

Bortz WM 2nd, Wallace DH, Wiley D. Sexual function in 1,202 ageing males: differentiating aspects. *J Gerontol A Biol Sci Med Sci* 1999; **54**: M237–41.

Carpenter CCJ, Mayer KH, Stein MD, *et al*. HIV infection in North American Women: Experience with 200 cases and a review of the literature. *Medicine* 1991; **70**: 307–25.

Catania JA, Stall R, Coates T, *et al*. Issues in AIDS primary prevention for middle aged and elderly Americans. *Generations* 1989; **13**: 50–4.

Centres for Disease Control and Prevention. *HIV/AIDS surveillance report* 1999; **11**: 16.

Centres for Disease Control and Prevention. Diagnosis and reporting of HIV and AIDS in States with HIV/AIDS surveillance. *MMWR* 2002; **51**: 595–9.

Ferro S, Salit IE. HIV infections in patients over 55 years of age. *J Acquir Immune Defic Syndr Hum Retrovirol* 1992; **5**: 348–53.

Fidel PL Jr, Sobel JD. Immunopathogenesis of recurrent vulvo-vaginal candidiasis. *Clinic Microbiol Rev* 1996; **9**: 335–48.

Gott CM. Sexual activity and risk-taking in later life. *Health Soc Care Community* 2001; **9**: 72–8.

Gott CM, Rogstad KE, Riley V, Ahmed-Jushuf I. Delay in symptom presentation among a sample of older GUM clinic attendees. *Int J STD AIDS* 1999; **10**: 43–6.

Hankins C, Coutllee F, Lapointe N, *et al*. Persistence of human papilloma virus (HPV) infection and HIV positive and negative women. Abstract presented at the *12th World AIDS Conference, Geneva, Switzerland, 1998* (Abstract 22303).

Health Protection Agency. *Diagnoses of selected STIs, by region, age and sex seen at GUM clinics, updated July 2004. National Level summary tables, 1995–2003*. London: Health Protection Agency, 2004. http://www.hpa.org.uk/infections/topics_az/hiv_and_sti/epidemiology/sti_data_1995-2003.pdf (last accessed 9 September 2004).

Lieber R. HIV in older Americans: an epidemiological perspective. *J Midwifery Women's Health* 2000; **45**: 176–82.

Maiman M, Fruchter RG, Serur E, *et al*: Recurrent cervical intraepithelial neoplasia in HIV seropositive women. *Obstet Gynecol* 1993; **82**: 170–4.

Moore LW, Ambergey LB. Older adults and HIV. *Assoc Oper Room Nurs J* 2000; **71**: 873–6.

Palefsky JM, Minkoff H, Kalish LA, *et al*. Cervicovaginal human papilloma virus infection in human immunodeficiency virus-1 positive and high risk HIV negative women. *J Natl Cancer Inst* 1999; **91**: 226–36.

Patterson B, Landay A, Anderson J, *et al*. Repertoire of chemokine receptor expression in the female genital tract: progesterone increases CCR5, CXCR4, and CCR3 expression. Abstract presented at the *12th World AIDS Conference, Geneva, Switzerland, 1998* (Abstract 21109).

Sharma R, Pickering J, McCormack WM. Trichomoniasis in a postmenopausal women cured after discontinuation of estrogen replacement therapy. *Sex Transm Dis* 1997; **24**: 543–4.

Sonnex C. Influence of ovarian hormones on urogenital infection. *Sex Transm Infect* 1998; **74**: 119.

van Benthem BH, Vernazza P, Coutinho RA, Prins M; European study on the natural history of HIV infection in women and the Swiss HIV cohort study. The impact of pregnancy and menopause on CD4 lymphocyte counts in HIV-infected women. *AIDS* 2002; **6**: 919–24.

Whipple B, Scura KW. The overlooked epidemic: HIV in older adults. *Am J Nurs* 1996; **96**: 23–8.

9 Male sexual function and its problems

Phillip Hodson

Introduction
Male sexual function
Effects of ageing
Disorders of desire
Erectile dysfunction
Disorders of ejaculation
Disorders of orgasm
Priapism
Conclusion

Introduction

Sexual health is very much a 'couple phenomenon' and thus the role of the male must be assessed. It is important to understand that men have different sexual expectations from women and are more likely to use pornography and sex aids. Men are more anxious about their sexual prowess and performance than most women. As one of the female characters in a Woody Allen book says, 'Sex without love is an empty experience.' 'Yes', replies Allen, 'but as empty experiences go it's one of the best.'

No one today thinks men and women are emotionally identical. John Gray's best-seller *Men are from Mars Women are from Venus* has made this extremely clear. Box 9.1 shows psychologist Oliver James' summing up of the differences.

For most men, therefore, sexuality is a highly rated aspect of their quality of life, and impairment can cause disharmony within the couple. Sexual dysfunction affects 31% of men, with the most common problem being erectile dysfunction. More than 152 million men worldwide are estimated to have experienced erectile dysfunction in 1995, and this number is estimated to rise by 170 million, to approximately 322 million, by the year 2025. Other complaints include disorders of desire, ejaculation and orgasm, as well as failure of detumescence.

Box 9.1

Oliver James' summing up of the differences between men and women

---

Women
- Place less emphasis on sexual intercourse as a goal, are more faithful and have fewer partners
- Fantasise less about sex, are less sexually explicit in their fantasies and focus more on the build-up than on the climax

Men
- Value physical attractiveness more highly than women – whether it be for marriage, a date or casual sex
- Place a higher premium on sexual intercourse
- Are keener on the idea of casual sex and more indiscriminate when considering it, think more often about sex and are more unfaithful
- Fantasise about a greater variety of partners, masturbate more and are more explicit about sexual acts during fantasies

---

Male sexual function

Various classifications of the male sexual cycle exist; of these, the one focusing on the functional activities is probably the most relevant to clinical practice. The normal male sexual response cycle thus can be divided into five interrelated events that occur in a defined sequence: libido, erection, ejaculation, orgasm and detumescence. Although lack of sex drive is common to both sexes, the aetiologies and management are different (Box 9.2).

Males reach peak sexual capacity in the late teens. With advancing age, a gradual decrease in sexual responsiveness occurs; this is characterized by an

---

Box 9.2

Same problem, different solutions

- Men and women identify different points of friction when a relationship begins to fail
- Men are far more likely to see the difficulty as a technical hitch rather than a crisis
- When men stonewall, women generally escalate their demands for a more emotional response
- As a last resort, women tend to drag up every single past occasion on which a partner has failed to satisfy them
- Men interpret this as a declaration of war – often voting with their feet

---

increase of the time required to achieve full erection and a decrease in the effectiveness of psychic and tactile stimuli. The plateau phase is also prolonged, and the maintenance of erection requires continuing direct genital stimulation. Orgasm and the feeling of ejaculatory inevitability may become less intense. Penile detumescence occurs more rapidly, and the refractory period is more prolonged. The ejaculatory volume also decreases with age. It is not clear at present whether some of these changes are related to the age-associated decline in serum testosterone concentrations.

Effects of ageing

Relatively little research has been undertaken into sexuality in old age, but available surveys show that some form of sexual activity usually continues until the end of life. For example, in a sample of people aged 80–102 years, 62% of the men and 30% of the women were still having sexual intercourse. Sexual changes associated with ageing are:

- decreased frequency of activity
- decreased arousal in response to psychological stimuli
- decreased tactile sensitivity of penis
- increased refractory period after orgasm
- increased rates of erectile dysfunction with age
- decreased rates of premature ejaculation.

Disorders of desire

The Diagnostic and Statistical Manual-IV (DSM-IV) defined hypoactive sexual desire (HSD) as persistently or recurrently deficient (or absent) sexual fantasy and desire for sexual activity leading to marked distress or interpersonal difficulty. More than 15% of adult men are generally estimated to have HSD. The diagnosis of primary desire loss in men is one of exclusion. Factors known to affect sexual function include major psychological disorders, androgen deficiency, chronic medical conditions, drugs (such as antihypertensives) and substance abuse.

Psychological disorders include psychiatric illnesses and preoccupation with a life crisis or grief. Depression, anxiety and schizophrenia commonly are associated with reduced desire and arousal. Conversely, mania and hypomania can be accompanied by hypersexuality. Traumatic employment or marriage-related issues may contribute to diminished self-image and heightened anxiety, leading to male sexual dysfunction.

Patients with a primary neurological disease, such as epilepsy, parkinsonism and the after effects of a stroke, may have diminished sexual arousal. The pathogenesis of desire insufficiency in these disorders seems to

Table 9.1

Causes of male sexual dysfunction

Clinical presentation	Common causes
Disorders of desire	
Hypoactive sexual desire (HSD)	• Psychological (eg depression, marital discord) • CNS disease (partial epilepsy, Parkinson's, poststroke) • Androgen deficiency • Drugs (antihypertensives, antidepressants, antipsychotics, alcohol, narcotics, dopamine blockers, antiandrogens)
Erectile dysfunction	• Psychological • Drugs (antihypertensives, anticholinergics, antidepressants, antipsychotics, cigarette smoking, illicit drugs) • Systemic diseases (cardiac, hepatic, renal, diabetes, postorgan transplant, pelvic irradiation) • Androgen deficiency and other hormonal disturbance • Peripheral vascular disease • Neurological disease (Parkinson's, Alzheimer's) • Penile disease (Peyronie's, priapism, phimosis) • Iatrogenic (pelvic irradiation, spinal injury)
Disorders of ejaculation	
Premature ejaculation (primary or secondary)	• Psychogenic (neurotic personality, anxiety/depression, partner problems) • Organic (increased central dopaminergic activity, increased penile sensitivity)
Absent or retarded emission	• Sympathetic denervation (diabetes, surgical injury, irradiation) • Drugs (sympatholytics, CNS depressants) • Androgen deficiency
Orgasmic dysfunction	• Drugs (selective serotonin reuptake inhibitors, tricyclic antidepressants, monoamine oxidase inhibitors, illicit drugs) • Neurological disease (multiple sclerosis, Parkinson's) • Psychogenic (performance anxiety, hypoactive)
Failure of detumescence	
Structural penile disease	• Penile structural abnormalities (Peyronie's, phimosis)
Priapism	• Disease (sickle cell anaemia), drugs (intrapenile vasoactive injections)

CNS, central nervous system

be multifactorial in origin and includes disease-related hormone abnormalities, physical restrictions and reduced general well-being.

Many drugs can reduce libido, potentially leading to poor compliance and adverse health consequences. Helpful measures include delaying the dose until after sexual intercourse, taking a drug holiday at suitable times, reducing the dose or changing to another agent.

Erectile dysfunction

Erectile dysfunction (ED) is the consistent inability to achieve or maintain an erection for sexual performance and is a common condition. The MALES study, involving 27 839 men aged 20–75 years interviewed in eight countries (United States, United Kingdom, Germany, France, Italy, Spain, Mexico and Brazil), found an overall prevalence of approximately 16%. Prevalence of ED varied markedly by country, however – from a high of 22% in the USA to a low of 10% in Spain. Prevalence increases with age, with estimates ranging from 25–30% of men aged between 60 and 70 years in the surveys of Kinsey, Schiavi and colleagues in 1990 to 52% in the Massachusetts Male Aging Study, which was undertaken in men aged 40–70 years.

Men with comorbid medical conditions and risk factors, including cardiovascular disease, hypertension, dyslipidaemia and depression, all reported higher prevalence of ED (Table 9.1). Men with ED also reported increased prevalence rates of these comorbid conditions.

With regard to depression, in the cross-sectional Massachusetts Male Aging Study, the incidence of moderate to complete ED was estimated to be nearly 90%, 60% and 25% in men with severe, moderate and minimal depression, respectively.

Many commonly prescribed pharmacological agents, such as antihypertensives, anticholinergics (which are also found in non-prescription common cold cures and hypnotics), antidepressants and antipyschotics, can adversely influence sexual function. The percentage of men with complete ED in the Massachusetts Male Aging Study who were taking hypoglycaemic agents (26%), antihypertensives (14%), vasodilators (36%) and cardiac drugs (28%) was significantly higher than the 9.6% observed for the sample as a whole. The cause of ED may not always be related to the individual drugs but to the underlying disease. For example, ED occurs in about half of diabetic men, which is twice the incidence in their non-diabetic counterparts, and the frequency increases with age. Another possibility, as in the case of antihypertensives, is the reduction of blood pressure in the face of penile arterial atherosclerosis which leads to ED.

At present, it is not clear whether recreational or illicit drugs, such as alcohol, methadone and heroin, reduce sexual potency by influencing the secretion and metabolism of androgens or by causing general physical and psychological deterioration in the addict.

Smoking is a major risk factor for the development of erectile dysfunction. Smoking impairs erection through a variety of mechanisms, including atherosclerosis, reduction in testosterone production, inappropriate adrenergic stimulation and inhibition of local vasodilator release.

Erectile dysfunction can accompany a variety of acute and chronic neurological disease. Loss of erectile or ejaculatory functions in patients with spinal cord injuries depends on the level and extent of the damage. Upper motor neuron lesions diminish the erectile response to psychogenic stimuli but leave the reflexogenic erections intact. The degree of diminution in psychogenic erections is directly related to the extent of the lesion. In contrast, lower motor neuron lesions abolish the reflexogenic response without altering psychogenic erections, except when the lesion is complete.

Disorders of ejaculation

A spectrum of disorders of ejaculation exists, ranging from mild premature to severely retarded or absent ejaculation. Several surveys among different populations estimate its prevalence at 29%, with a range between 1% and 75% depending on the population and the defining criteria. The DSM-IV defines the diagnostic criteria for premature or rapid ejaculation as follows:

1. Persistent or recurrent ejaculation with minimum sexual stimulation that occurs before, upon or shortly after penetration and before either partner wishes it.
2. Marked distress or interpersonal difficulty.
3. The condition does not arise as a direct effect of substance abuse, ie opiate withdrawal.

Disorders of orgasm

Male orgasmic disorder is defined as a persistent or recurrent delay in, or absence of, orgasm after a normal sexual excitement phase during sexual activity. The disorder is relatively rare, occurring in 3–10% of patients who present with sexual dysfunction. Table 9.1 describes the most common causes of orgasmic dysfunction.

Priapism

Priapism is failure to detumesce within four hours. If it persists longer than 4–6 hours the danger of thrombosis, fibrosis and potentially gangrene increases considerably. Urgent treatment is critical.

Conclusion

It is important to realise that male sexual problems can have a major impact on a couple's relationship. The male agenda is vastly different from that of the woman. Although some problems are similar, the solutions are different.

Further reading

Allen W. *Love and death*. New York: Random House, 1979.

American Psychiatric Association. *Diagnostic and statistical manual of mental disorders (fourth edition)*. Washington: American Psychiatric Association, 1994.

Araujo AB, Durante R, Feldman HA, *et al*. The relationship between depressive symptoms and male erectile dysfunction: cross-sectional results from the Massachusetts Male Aging Study. *Psychosom Med* 1998; **60**: 458–65.

Ayta IA, McKinlay JB, Krane RJ. The likely worldwide increase in erectile dysfunction between 1995 and 2025 and some possible policy consequences. *Br J Urol Int* 1999; **84**: 50–6.

Bretschneider JG, McCoy NL. Sexual interest and behaviour in healthy 80-102 year olds. *Arch Sex Behav* 1988; **17**: 109–29.

Feldman HA, Goldstein I, Hatzichristou DG, *et al*. Impotence and its medical and psychosocial correlates: results of the Massachusetts Male Aging Study. *J Urol* 1994; **151**: 54–61

Gottman J. *Why marriages succeed or fail and how you can make yours last*. New York: Fireside, 1995.

Gray J. *Men are from Mars, women are from Venus*. New York: Harper Collins, 1993.

Gregoire A. ABC of sexual health: male sexual problems. *BMJ* 1999; **318**: 245–7.

James O. *They f*** you up your mum and dad: how to survive family life*. London: Bloomsbury, 1993.

Johnson AM, Wadsworth J, Wellings K, *et al*. *Sexual Attitudes and Lifestyles*. Oxford: Blackwell, 1994.

Kandeel FR, Koussa VK, Swerdloff RS. Male sexual function and its disorders: physiology, pathophysiology, clinical investigation, and treatment. *Endocr Rev* 2001; **22**: 342–88.

Laumann EO, Nicolosi A, Glasser DB, *et al*. Sexual problems among women and men aged 40-80 y: prevalence and correlates identified in the Global Study of Sexual Attitudes and Behaviors. *Int J Impot Res* 2004 advance online publication, 24 June.

Laumann EO, Paik A, Rosen RC. Sexual dysfunction in the United States: prevalence and predictors. *JAMA* 1999; **281**: 537–44.

Metz ME, Pryor JL, Nesvacil LJ, *et al*. Premature ejaculation: a psychophysiological review. *J Sex Marital Ther* 1997; **23**: 3–23.

Morley JE, Kaiser F, Raum WJ, *et al*. Potentially predictive and manipulable blood serum correlates of aging in the healthy human male: progressive decreases in bioavailable testosterone, dehydroepiandrosterone sulfate, and the ratio of insulin-like growth factor 1 to growth hormone. *Proc Natl Acad Sci USA* 1997; **94**: 7537–42.

Rosen RC, Fisher WA, Eardley I, *et al*. Men's Attitudes to Life Events and Sexuality

(MALES) Study. The multinational Men's Attitudes to Life Events and Sexuality (MALES) study: I. Prevalence of erectile dysfunction and related health concerns in the general population. *Curr Med Res Opin* 2004; **20**: 607–17.

Rosen MP, Greenfield AJ, Walter TG, *et al.* Cigarette smoking: an independent risk factor for atherosclerosis in the hypogastric-cavernous arterial bed of men with arteriogenic impotence. *J Urol* 1991; **145**: 759–63.

Rosen RC, Leiblum SR. Treatment of sexual disorders in the 1990s: an integrated approach. *J Consult Clin Psychol* 1995; **63**: 877–90.

Schiavi RC, Rehman J. Sexuality and aging. *Urol Clin North Am* 1995; **22**: 711–26.

Schiavi RC, Schreiner-Engel P, Mandeli J, *et al.* Healthy aging and male sexual function. *Am J Psychiatry* 1990; **147**: 766–71.

Walsh PC, Wilson JD. Impotence and infertility in men. In: Braunwald E, Isselbacher KJ, Petersdorf RS, *et al*, eds. *Harrison's principals of internal medicine*. New York: McGraw-Hill, 1987: 217–20.

10 Coping with male problems

Clive Gingell

Introduction
Erectile dysfunction
Benign enlargement of the prostate
Prostate cancer
The future

Introduction

The main problems of concern are symptoms due to erectile dysfunction (ED) and prostatic enlargement with age – either benign or malignant. Erectile dysfunction affects a relationship and may cause considerable frustration if the female partner wishes to remain sexually active. Both conditions are age-related and eminently treatable. Erectile dysfunction may result '*de novo*' due to a man's age and comorbidities, doubling with each decade over 50, but it may be associated with prostate problems. Indeed, when symptomatic benign prostatic hyperplasia (BPH) and ED coexist, combination therapy with an α-blocker and a phosphodiesterase type 5 (PDE5) inhibitor can be extremely effective. Men, however, are much less likely than women to consult health professionals, but they can, albeit reluctantly, be persuaded by their partners to seek advice.

Erectile dysfunction

Erectile dysfunction is the consistent inability to achieve or maintain an erection for sexual performance and is a common condition that affects 16% of adult men (Chapter 9). It is increasingly common with advancing years and is enhanced by comorbidities often present in the ageing male, such as vascular disease, hypertension and diabetes, as well as a variety of medications (Chapter 9). In the MALES study, among men who reported ED, 58% had actively sought medical attention for their condition; however, only 16% of men with ED were currently being treated with oral PDE5 therapy.

Management

It is possible from a treatment point of view to modify adverse lifestyle factors, such as smoking, alcohol intake and substance abuse. Antihypertensive medication can be altered, sometimes with a beneficial result. Other common medications associated with ED are antidepressants and antipsychotics. Psychosocial factors, such as relationship issues, stress and depression itself must also be addressed. A thorough medical and sexual history is fundamental and must include the patient's medication. The clinical examination should involve inspection and palpitation of the genitalia and blood pressure, peripheral pulses and urine tests. Measurement of the plasma testosterone is also advisable, and, indeed, is often requested by the patient. Total testosterone, although the most common measure clinically, does not yield meaningful information about tissue androgen exposure because of its binding to sex hormone binding globulin (SHBG). Free testosterone measurements are more reliable but are not routinely available, so the free androgen index (testosterone/SHBG × 100) is used more frequently but is not totally reliable. Any adjustments to lifestyle, such as weight loss, cessation of smoking and alteration of blood pressure, are worth pursuing.

Therapy

The licensing of the first effective oral therapy, sildenafil, in 1998, and the subsequent development of other oral and sublingual drugs, has been a major breakthrough in the treatment of ED and has had a profound effect on the management of this condition.

Oral phosphodiesterase inhibitors

Sildenafil, tadalafil and vardenafil are phosphodiesterase type 5 (PDE5) inhibitors that prevent the inactivation of cyclic guanosine monophosphate (cGMP), the most important intracellular secondary messenger, causing relaxation of the smooth muscle cell and allowing an erection to take place.

Taken orally, they enhance the normal erectile mechanism and are very specific in their effect, with an excellent side-effect profile. The most common complications are headache, facial flushing, heartburn and nasal congestion, with occasional muscle aches with tadalafil. Sexual stimulation is necessary for an effect to occur, but absorption of sildenafil (not vardenafil or tadalafil) can be delayed by having had a fatty meal.

PDE5 inhibitors can be used safely to treat ED in patients with coronary artery disease, previous myocardial infarction, coronary artery bypass surgery and stable angina, except in those taking nitrates or nicorandil, as coadministration can result in a significant drop in blood pressure.

The usual starting dose in most patients is:

- **Sildenafil**: 50mg, increasing to 100 mg if necessary, especially in diabetics

- **Tadalafil**: 10–20 mg and **vardenafil** 10–20 mg are both rapidly absorbed, although tadalafil gives a longer period of responsiveness (up to 36 hours post-dosing), enabling greater freedom for the timing of sexual activity.

Many so-called PDE5 failures are due to lack of appropriate instructions and counselling by the prescribing doctor and not to the lack of efficacy of the drug itself.

Sublingual apomorphine

This sublingual formulation of apomorphine with controlled absorption has excellent bioavailability through the oral mucosa, and erections may occur in as little as 10 minutes. The most common side-effect is mild to moderate nausea in 3–4% of patients. It is optimally suited to those with mild to moderate ED of primary psychogenic aetiology. Sequential administration enhances the effect, so if the first dose does not work, the patient should not give up but should try again. There is no interaction between apomorphine and other drugs, so it can therefore be given to patients who cannot be weaned off nitrates. The success rate is less than 50%.

Non-oral methods

Intracavernosal injections – prostaglandin E_1 (PGE1, eg alprostadil) is usually very successful, but many men find penile self-injection off-putting. In non-responders to PGE1, combination therapy with PGE1 and papaverine, together with 1 or 2mg phentolamine can prove to be effective in the motivated patient. A third successful injection is a combination of phentolamine and vasoactive intestinal peptide, which does not have the alprostadil ache and is preferred by many patients.

Medicated urethral system for erections (MUSE) – a small pellet of intraurethral PGE1 is a more attractive proposition to many patients than an intrapenile injection, although it only succeeds in 50% of patients.

Mechanical devices – in those patients who do not respond to other therapy, vacuum constriction devices can be offered. It is critical that the patients are properly instructed in their use. They work, whatever the underlying cause of ED, by producing an erection with sufficient rigidity for penetration. They seem to be most suited for the older man in a long-term, durable relationship, who does not respond to pharmacological treatment and does not wish to proceed to surgery

Surgery – the insertion of either a malleable or inflatable penile prosthesis is a valid option in motivated patients who do not respond to more conservative measures. A major concern for patients and surgeons remains – prosthesis infection. Corrective surgery is also required in men with penile curvature secondary to Peyronie's disease, where the degree of curvature is such that it prevents penetration.

Benign enlargement of the prostate

Over 40% of men over 60 years of age experience moderate-to-severe lower urinary tract symptoms (LUTS). These symptoms are usually due to benign prostatic hyperplasia (BPH) causing bladder outlet obstruction and can have a major impact on quality of life. Box 10.1 contains key facts about this condition. Dihydrotestosterone (DHT), produced from testosterone via the 5α-reductase isoenzymes (type 1 and 2), is the primary androgen responsible for the development of BPH. Prostatic-specific antigen (PSA) is a strong predictor of progression.

The urinary symptom complex of urgency, frequency, hesitancy, poor flow and terminal dribbling adversely affects the quality of life. Lower urinary tract symptoms impose restrictions on day trips together, bus journeys, holidays and many other social gatherings. The main disruption to a man's partner caused by prostatic enlargement is nocturnal frequency resulting in sleep disturbance. It is truly a 'couple's' problem.

Management

The medical management of LUTS due to BPH has advanced considerably. Two classes of medication with different mechanisms of action are available for its treatment.

Box 10.1

Key points about benign enlargement of the prostate

- Prostate volume increases with time and a volume >30 cm^3 increases the risk of acute retention three-fold
- Prostate-specific antigen is a strong predictor of BPH progression
- Within four years, 10% of patients with BPH will require surgical intervention, and men who present with acute retention are at higher risk of developing complications than men who undergo elective prostatectomy
- If a 60 year-old man survives until he is 80 years old, he has a 23% probability of experiencing acute retention
- Men aged over 60 years with an enlarged prostate and obstructive symptoms have a 39% lifetime risk of surgery
- The risk of acute retention is increased four-fold in patients with urinary flow of <12 ml/second

Alpha-blockers

These are effective in alleviating LUTS. They act on the stromal smooth muscle of the prostate, improving flow of urine. Although more uroselective sustained release α-blockers, such as alfusosin and tamsulosin, have been developed recently, none affects either the composition or size of the prostate gland.

Specific inhibitors of the enzyme 5α-reductase

Specific inhibitors of the enzyme 5α-reductase, which metabolizes testosterone into the more potent androgen dihydrotestosterone (DHT), do reduce prostate size. Finasteride reduces DHT by approximately 70% and improves the urinary flow rate, lowering the risk of acute retention, and therefore the need for surgery, by more than 50%. Dutasteride is an inhibitor of both type I and type II 5 α-reductase and has been shown to reduce serum DHT by more than 90%. It also significantly reduces the risk of both acute retention and elective surgery, as well as improving the patient's symptoms and flow rates. It can be prescribed on its own or in combination with an α-blocker. It may take up to six months for either of the 5α-reductase inhibitors to be fully effective. Both reduce the serum concentration of prostatic cancer markers, such as PSA, and both may cause loss of desire.

Desmopressin

Desmopressin, 0.2 mg at night, can be very effective in the management of many cases of nocturnal frequency. In other patients, the very early evening administration of a quick-acting diuretic to get rid of oedema accumulated during the daytime will reduce nocturnal frequency considerably.

Prostate cancer

Prostate cancer is the most common cancer found in elderly men in the UK. It affects around 22,000 men in Britain and has an annual incidence of 20 men per 100,000 and a mortality of 15 per 100,000, with approximately 10,000 deaths each year. The incidence has been rising steadily over the past 30 years, due, in part, to an ever-increasing ageing population but also to the more widespread use of PSA testing. This has resulted in earlier diagnosis of the disease process, allowing the potential of curative therapy, but treatment with radical prostatectomy, conformal external beam radiotherapy or brachytherapy carries with it an increased risk of impotence. The introduction of nerve-sparing radical retropubic prostatectomy (NSRRP) aims to preserve erectile function.

An alternative option of lowering the serum testosterone level, by medical castration with an luteinizing hormone-releasing hormone (LHRH) analogue, also results in loss of desire. The non-steroidal antiandrogens, such as bicalutamide, prevent binding of testosterone and its more potent metabolite 5HT, to androgen receptors in the prostate, and libido is preserved. The excess circulating testosterone, however, is converted by aromatase inhibition to an oestrogenic compound and therefore painful gynaecomastia can occur. This can be controlled by pre-treatment radiotherapy to the breasts.

Small volume, localized, well-differentiated carcinoma of the prostate (often detected in a few 'chips' after transurethral resection of a benign prostate) can be managed expectantly. Such patients, especially those aged over 70 years with comorbidity, are particularly suited to a 'watchful waiting' approach by regular review and PSA monitoring. Hormone manipulation, because of the side-effects, can be deferred often for many years. Many such patients die with their disease and not from it. It is important for the man's wife or partner to be involved in the decision-making process and to be given a realistic prognosis.

In a man who presents with locally advanced disease that is metastatic in the bony skeleton, it has to be accepted that the mortality is about 50% at two years. It is likely that there is a population of hormone-resistant cells within any prostate cancer that continues to multiply and progress despite hormonal treatment.

The future

There is much clinical interest and considerable research activity in developing effective local applications of vasoactive agents to the penis to produce good quality erections without systemic side-effects in the patient or his partner. Locally applied, rapidly absorbed preparations will probably have a role to play. Combination therapy has to date not been studied extensively. The potential of using centrally acting drugs and peripherally acting agents delivered orally in combination with locally applied preparations in the more clinically challenging patient is potentially an exciting therapeutic opportunity. Much has already been achieved in the field of andrological research and it is highly likely that further preparations will become available in the very near future. It is important that general practitioners overcome their inhibitions and question their patients about their sex lives, particularly in the presence of common predisposing factors, including cardiovascular disease, hypertension, diabetes, depression and the use of a variety of medications.

Further reading

Atiemo HO, Szostak MJ, Sklar GN. Salvage of sildenafil failures referred from primary care physicians. *J Urol* 2003; **170**: 2356–8.

Bar-Chama N, Zaslau S, Gribetz M. Intracavernosal injection therapy and other treatment options for erectile dysfunction. *Endocr Pract* 1997; 3: 54–9.

Drugs and Therapeutics Bulletin. New oral drugs for erectile dysfunction. *Drug Ther Bull* 2004; **42**: 49–52.

Eisenberger M, Partin A. Progress toward identifying aggressive prostate cancer. *N Engl J Med* 2004; **351**: 180–1.

Fiet J, Giton F, Fidaa I, *et al.* Development of a highly sensitive and specific new testosterone time-resolved fluoroimmunoassay in human serum. *Steroids* 2004; **69**: 461–71.

Garraway WM, Russell EB, Lee RJ, *et al.* Impact of previously unrecognised benign prostatic hyperplasia on the daily activities of middle-aged and elderly men. *Br J Gen Pract* 1993; **43**: 318–21.

Hatzichristou DG, Apostolidis A, Beckos A, *et al.* Sildenafil failures may be due to inadequate instructions and follow up: a study of 100 non-responders. *Int J Impot Res* 2001; **13 (suppl)**: 4352.

Kirby RS, Christmas TJ, Brawer MK. *Prostate cancer.* St Louis: Mosby International, 2001.

Jackson G. Treatment of erectile dysfunction in patients with cardiovascular disease: guide to drug selection. *Drugs* 2004; **64**: 1533–45.

Jackson G, Keltai M, Gillies H, *et al.* Viagra is well tolerated by subjects with stable angina and erectile dysfunction during incremental treadmill exercise. *Eur Urol* 2002; **1** (suppl): 15.

Klee GG, Heser D. Techniques to measure testosterone in the elderly. *Mayo Clinic Proceedings* 2000; **75**: S19–25.

Oefelein MG, Agarwal PK, Resnick MI. Survival of patients with hormone refractory prostate cancer in the prostate specific antigen era. *J Urol* 2004; **171**: 1525–8.

O'Leary M. Erectile dysfunction. *Clin Evid* 2002; **(8)**: 872–80.

Pickard R, Emberton M, Neal DE. The management of men with acute urinary retention. *Br J Urol* 1998; **81**: 712–20.

Rosen RC, Fisher WA, Eardley I, *et al.* Men's Attitudes to Life Events and Sexuality (MALES) Study. The multinational Men's Attitudes to Life Events and Sexuality (MALES) study: I. Prevalence of erectile dysfunction and related health concerns in the general population. *Curr Med Res Opin* 2004; **20**: 607–17.

Schultheiss D. Regenerative medicine in andrology: tissue engineering and gene therapy as potential treatment options for penile deformations and erectile dysfunction. *Eur Urol* 2004; **46**: 162–9.

Seftel AD, Wilson SK, Knapp PM, *et al.* The efficacy and safety of tadalafil in United States and Puerto Rican men with erectile dysfunction. *J Urol* 2004; **172**: 652–7.

Smith RP, Malkowicz SB, Whittington R, *et al.* Identification of clinically significant prostate cancer by prostate-specific antigen screening. *Arch Intern Med* 2004; **164**: 1227–30.

Tubaro A, La Vecchia C; Uroscreening Study Group. The relation of lower urinary tract symptoms with life-style factors and objective measures of benign prostatic enlargement and obstruction: an Italian survey. *Eur Urol* 2004; **45**: 767–72.

Index

Page numbers in *italic* indicate boxes, figures and tables.